Who are Valerie and John Thompson and what *are* they doing sitting in a redwood hot tub in the middle of a pine grove?

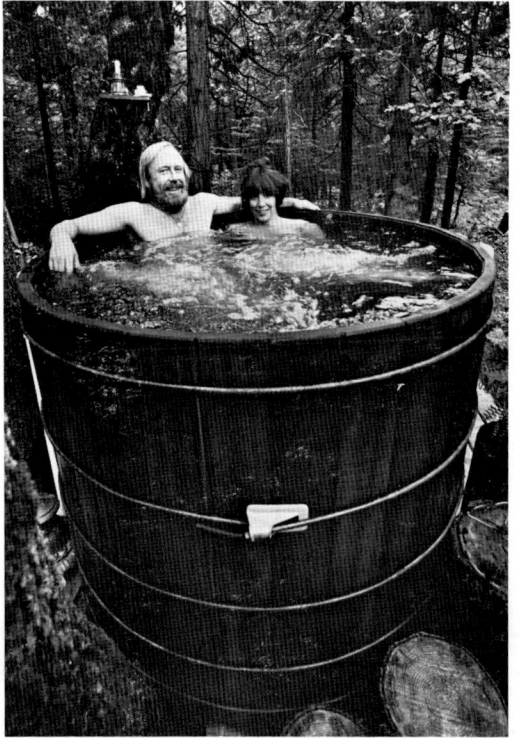

The Thompsons, actually, are a lot like the rest of us: pursued-by-mortgage-payments; making-ends-meet; traffic-jammed; nerve-racked. *Except* that they have, for at least an hour a day, escaped the breakneck speed at which most of us live our lives. Many of us are simply working too hard.

They got their hot tub under doctor's orders for Val's circulatory problems. What they found was that the hot tub changed their lives. There was something about sitting quietly in nature, in water heated to 105°F., that was *deeply* relaxing. But when they looked around for a book to tell them how to care for the tub and keep it going—and also something about the *manners* of communal bathing—they couldn't find it. So they researched it and wrote it and here it is: The Thompsons' Guide to How-Much-Does-One-Cost? A Tour of Sites; How-to-Backwash-the-Filter; So What About Bathing Suits?

CANNIBAL SOUP is offered with the hope that its warmth will reach deep into the weary bones of a nation that's earned a moment of peace, friendliness and relaxation. Imagine, an oasis in your own backyard....

CANNIBAL SOUP
TUBBING WITH THE THOMPSONS

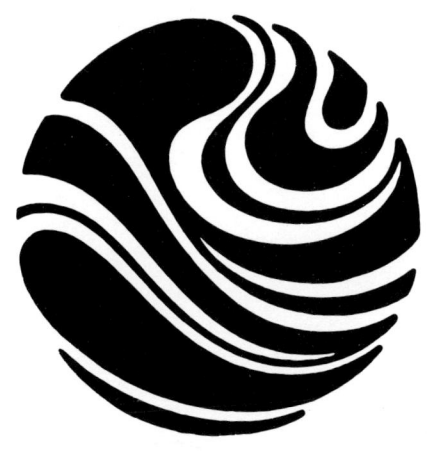

Valerie and John Thompson

photography by
George D. Lepp

A Prism Edition

To Duane Newcomb, for "The Newcomb Method" which gave us the courage to begin this book; and, to Dick Sutphen, for Tape P-207, which gave us the creative energy to complete it.

Cover and book design by Brenton Beck of Fifth Street Design Associates.

Copyright © 1978 by Valerie and John Thompson. All rights reserved.

A Prism Edition
Chronicle Books
870 Market Street
San Francisco, CA 94102

Library of Congress Cataloging in Publication Data

Thompson, John, 1936-
    Cannibal soup.

    1. Baths, Hot. 2. Bathing customs. I. Thompson, Valerie, 1942-   joint author. II. Title
RM822.H68T45 613'.41 78-1758

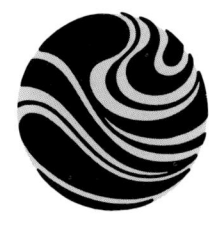

CONTENTS

1. IN THE BEGINNING 9

2. A QUICK DIP INTO THE HISTORY OF BATHING 15

3. THE RENAISSANCE OF THE HOT TUB 25

4. HOT TUB MYTHS AND FANTASIES 39

5. THROW THOSE SLEEPING PILLS AWAY 53

6. M-M-M-M-M-M-M-M-M-M-M 59

7. IF YOU'VE SEEN ONE, HAVE YOU SEEN THEM *ALL?* 71

8. TO DECK OR NOT TO DECK? 79

9. THE PARTS OF YOUR TUB THAT NOBODY SEES 87

THE THOMPSONS'
HOT TUB MAINTENANCE MANUAL 101
YOUR HOT TUB'S FIRST DAYS HOME
CHEMICALS
GENERAL OPERATING INSTRUCTIONS
TO CLEAN THE STRAINER BASKET
TO CLEAN THE FILTER
TO DRAIN THE TUB
TO RESTART THE TUB
HOW YOUR HOT TUB SAVES WATER AND POWER

ACKNOWLEDGEMENTS 107

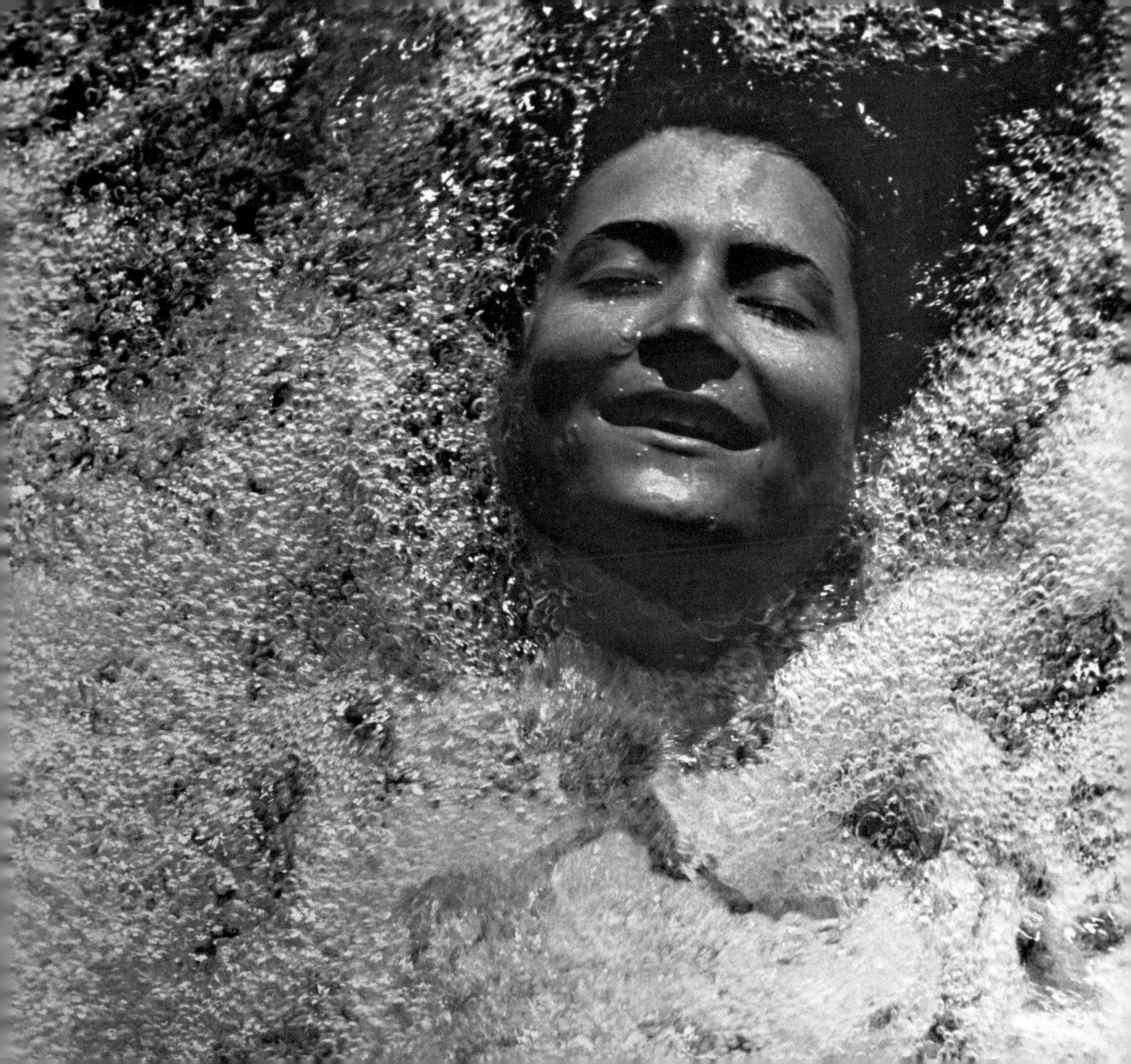

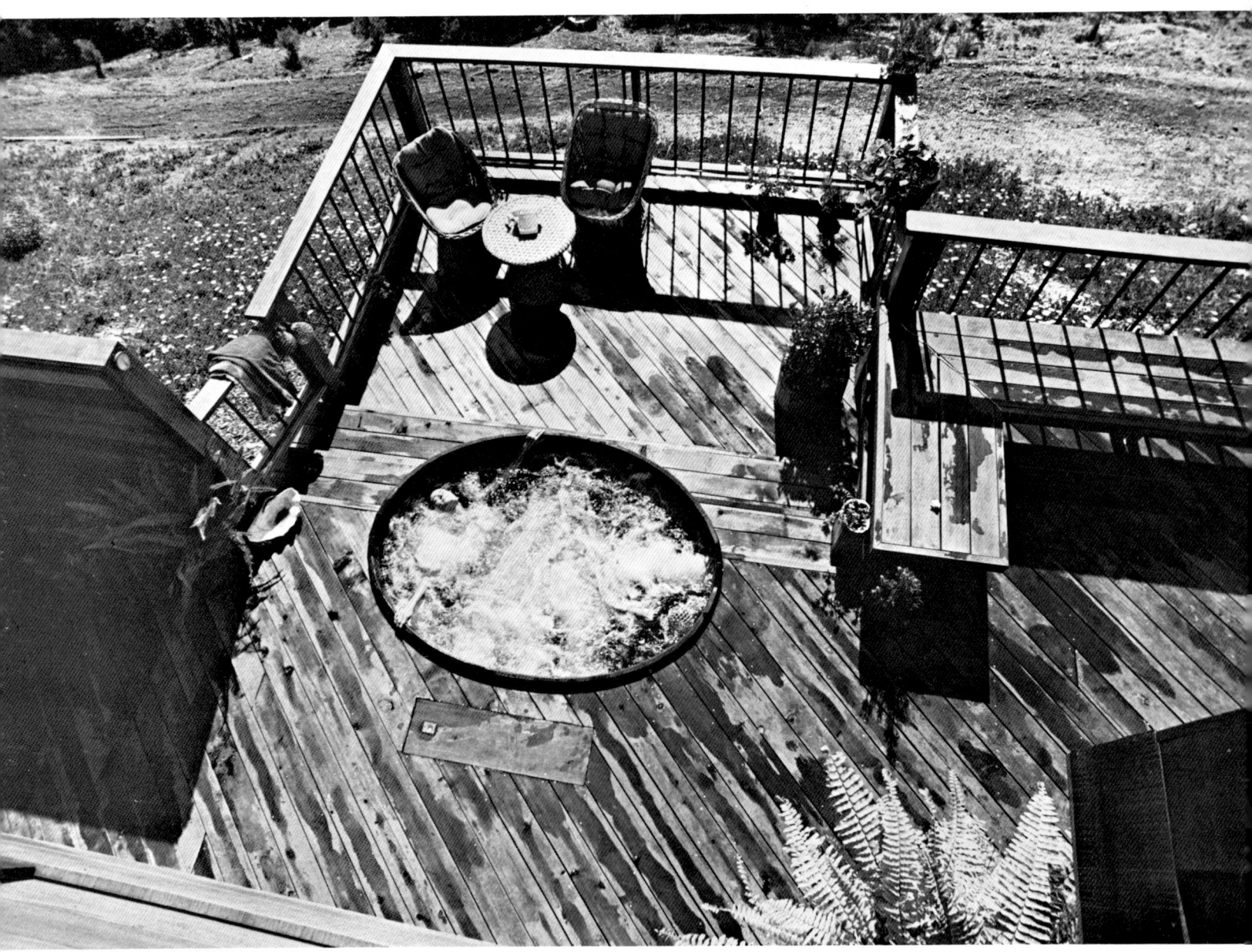

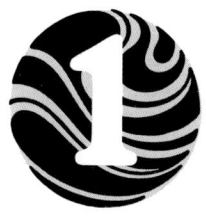

IN THE BEGINNING

"What *is* a hot tub?" Only last year, we too, asked that question. Almost overnight, the hot tub phenomenon has swept the country, beginning on the West Coast. We became acquainted with hot tubs when Valerie's doctor suggested that it might aid her circulation problem. At that time dealers were hard to find. Now, dealers proliferate, and hot tub ads decorate the pages of magazines as diverse as *New West, Penthouse, The New Yorker, Sunset* and *Rolling Stone.*

We're just two of the thousands of people who have discovered and embraced the redwood Jacuzzi—and have been introduced to a new way of life. As with all new products, there is a real need for a definitive manual to describe the product and its workings. This was especially true of the hot tub, because when we purchased ours, the dealer couldn't provide any written material aside from the manufacturer's warranties on the equipment. And after it was constructed, filled and the salesman left, we sat blissfully soaking in our brand-new acquisition, and suddenly realized that all his oral instructions had evaporated—rising like steam above our heads. *How often were we supposed to backwash the filter? In what order were the switches to be operated? Where were the instructions for the PH test kit?* We spent so much time making calls to the dealer for help, that we decided to compile all our notes and put them together in a book to make life a little easier for novice soakers.

So we found ourselves faced with the awesome task of writing the Hot Tub Bible—with the major drawback that we were just two average hot tub owners and couldn't count on one speck of divine guidance. But we entered into this with good will, enthusiasm and the sincere hope that you will find this book a help and an inspiration to enjoy many hours of healthy, relaxed and carefree tubbing.

While working on this book we had the pleasure of meeting and photographing many hot tubbers in

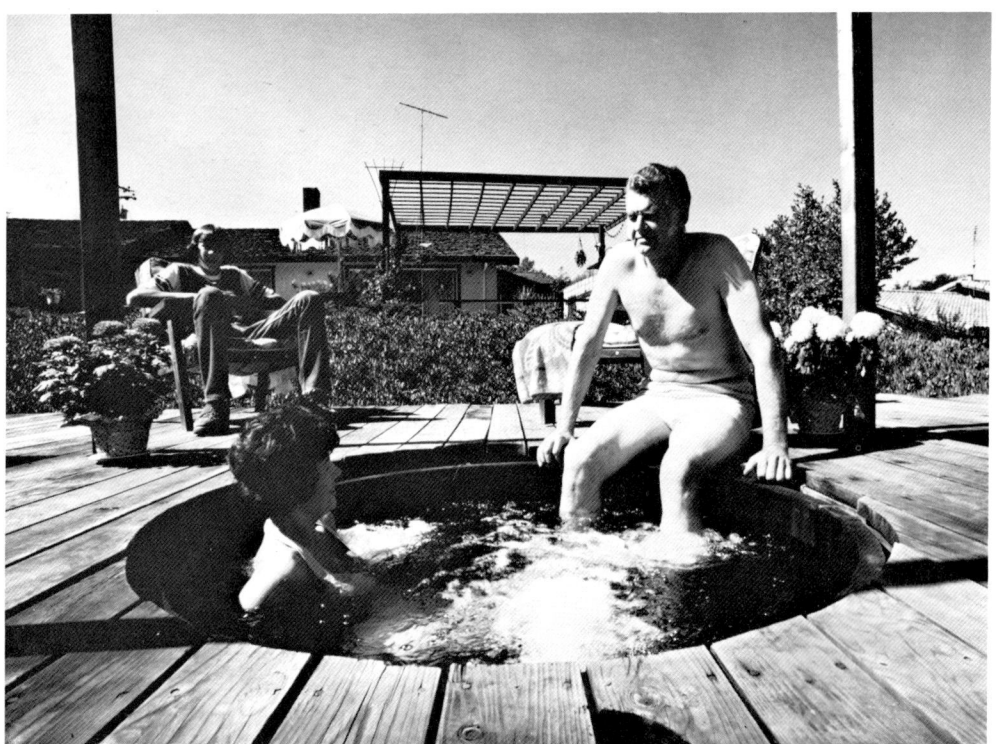

Athletes do it; little boys and girls do it; moms and dads and babies do it too. Hot tubs seem to tickle everybody pink.

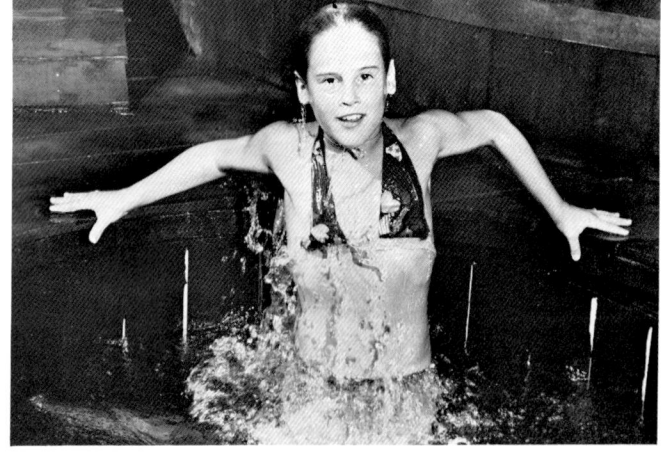

their tubs. One fact frequently struck us—we found the hot tub owners were very busy people. One tubber scheduled our interview around an exhibit of her paintings; another was busily preparing for a horse show. At one interview, two young track stars were soaking away their aches and pains when we arrived.

Instead of the "laid-back hippies" we had half-expected to find, we discovered vivacious, vigorous people using the tub as a means of keeping physically fit. Bicyclers, backpackers and joggers told us about soothing their sore calves by soaking in the tub after miles of strenuous exertion. One career

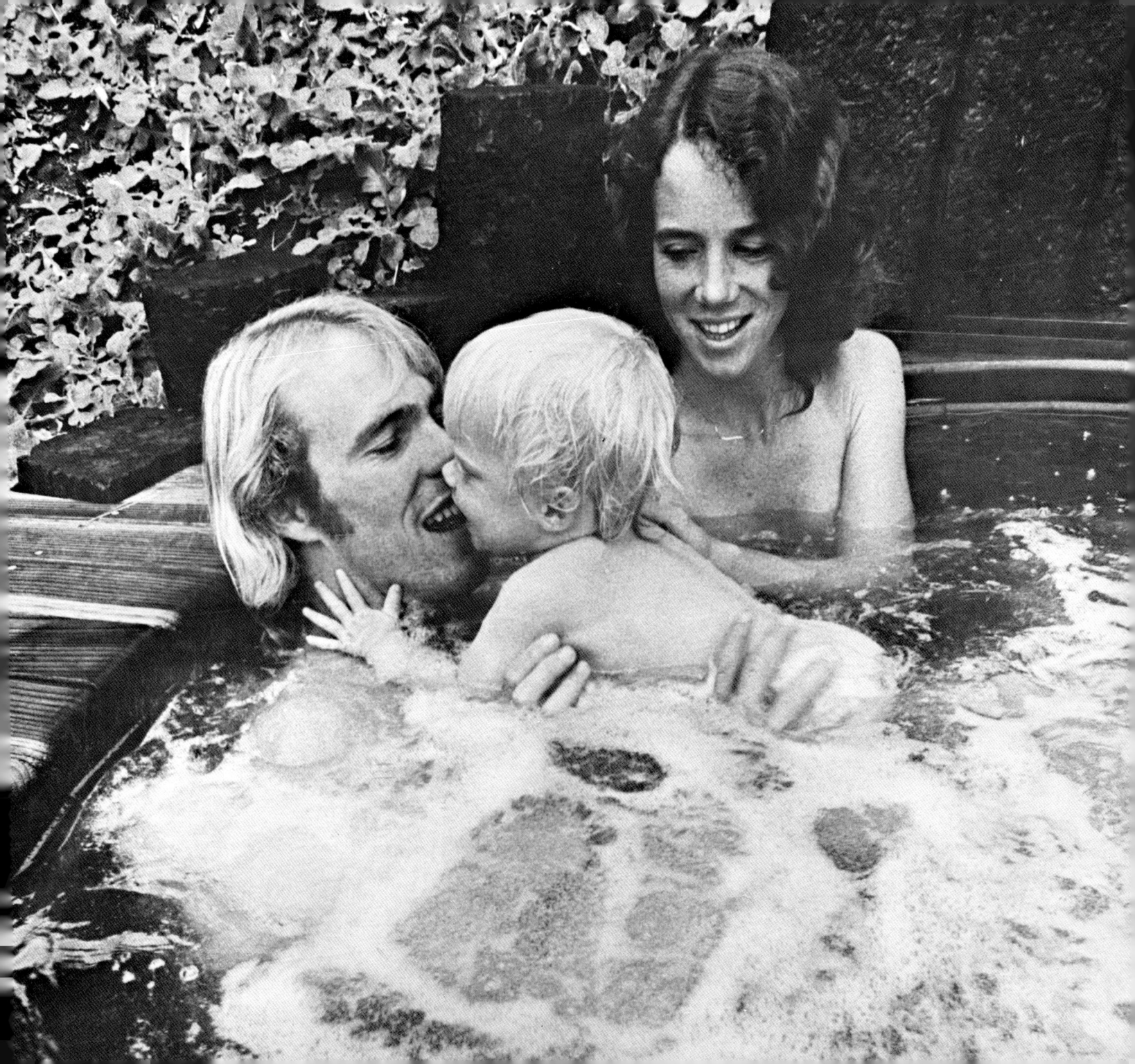

CANNIBAL SOUP

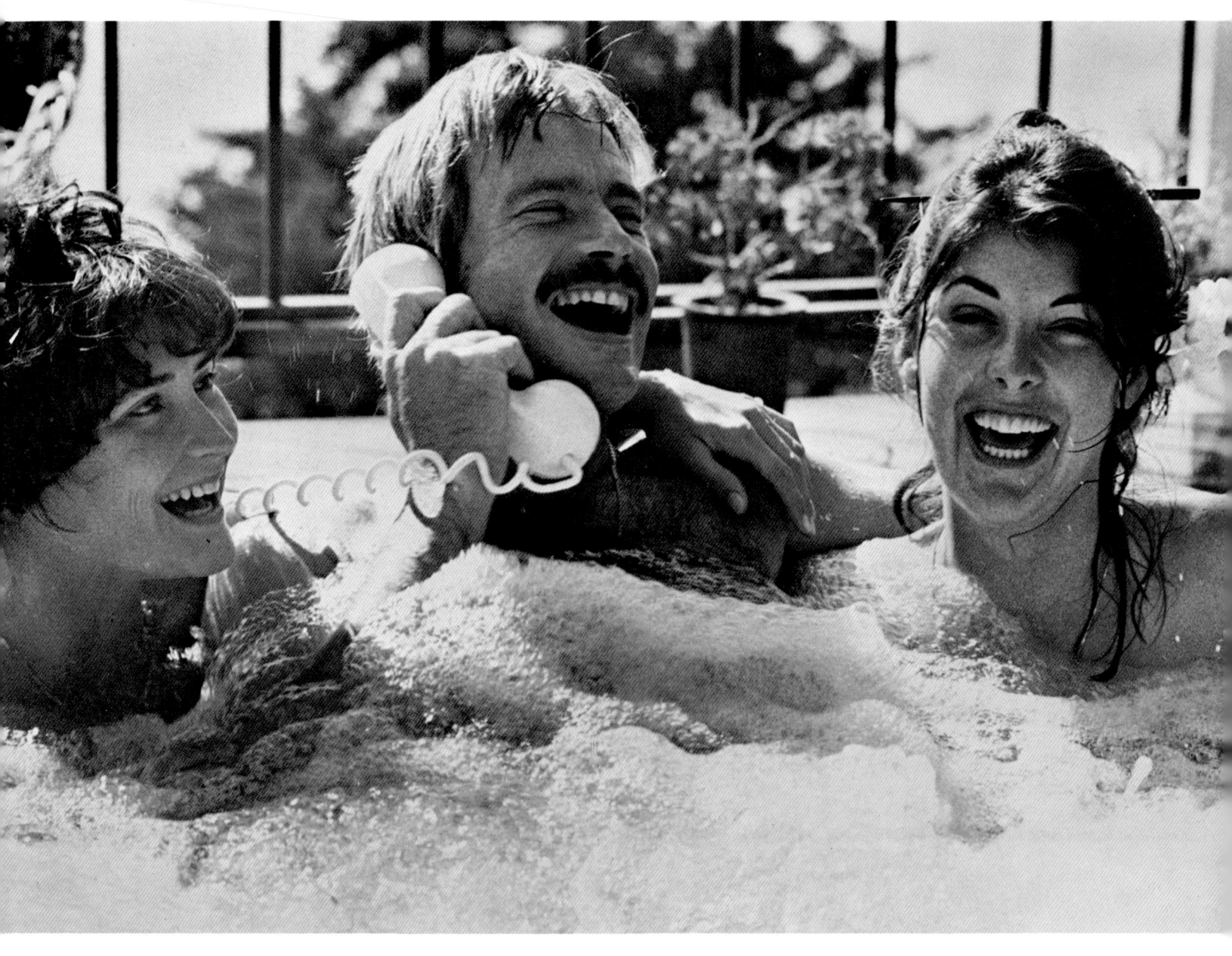

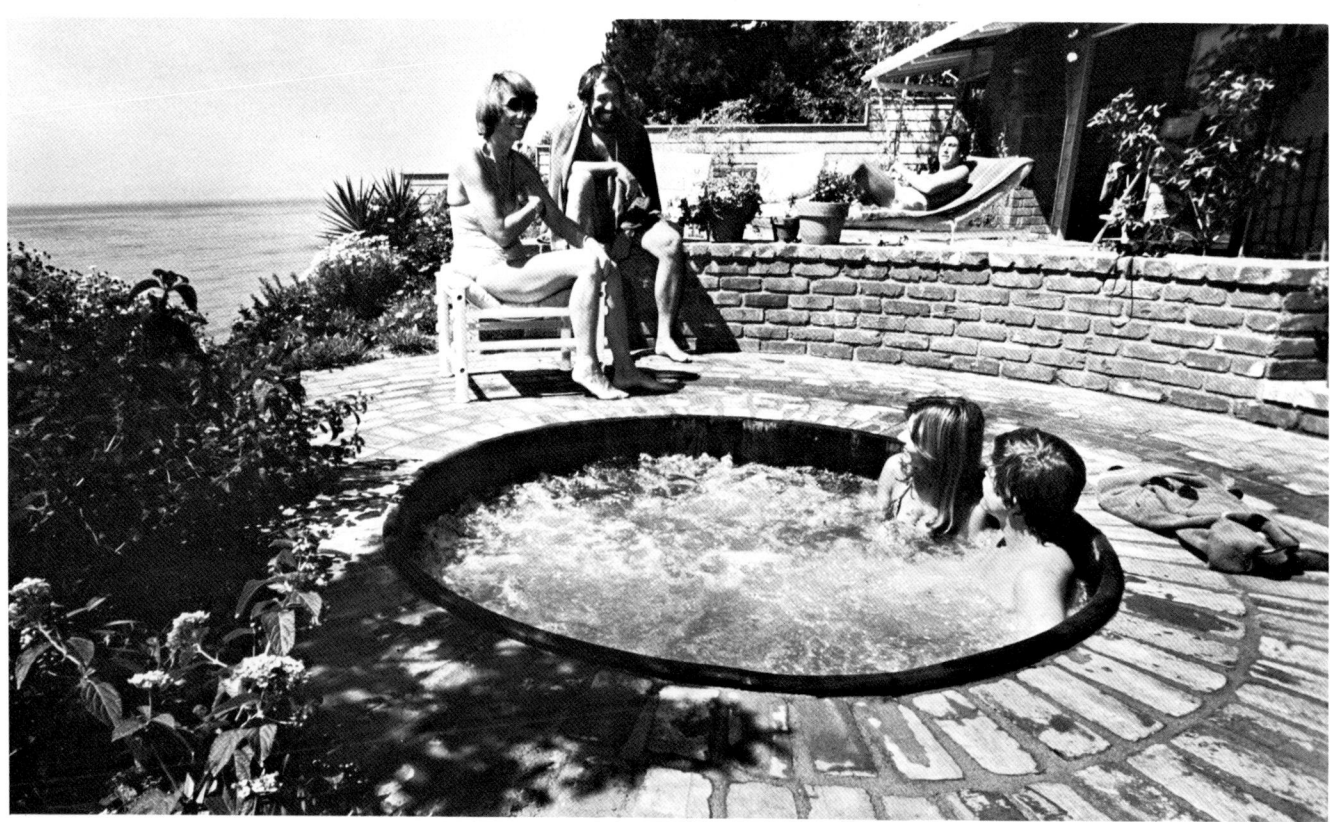

woman said, "Instead of taking a Valium, I plunk into the hot tub! After awhile I'm ready for anything!" We talked to a pressured businessman who reads *The Wall Street Journal* while up to his neck in the massaging bubbles of his tub. He says the edges of his paper get a bit damp, but that it's a small price to pay for relaxation.

We met people in the best of health; we met people with bad backs, fractured ankles, swollen legs, and chronic headaches. All attested to the wonderful benefits of the hot tub. A sprightly lady in her seventies who exercises daily in her tub said, "It is exactly what the doctor ordered!"

We met tubbers who have full-time jobs yet make time for painting, growing orchids or exotic bamboo, photography, woodcarving, fishing, snowshoeing, skiing, or ballet. We didn't find one lazy soul in the bunch! Everyone was interesting to talk to, full of energy, and—above all—they *seemed* to be happy. How much of this aura of well-being can be credited to the hot tub we can't presume to say, but they do *smile* a lot.

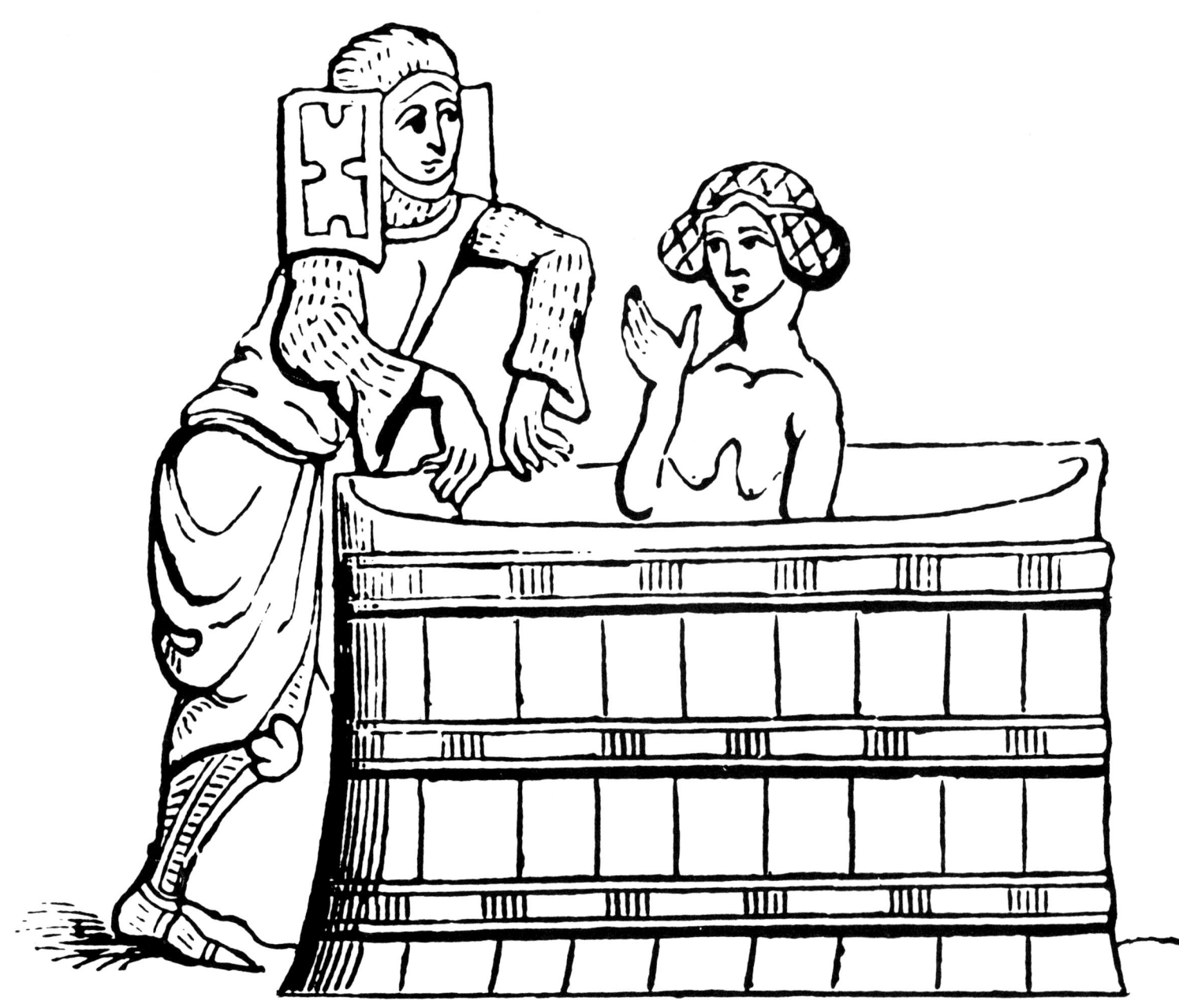

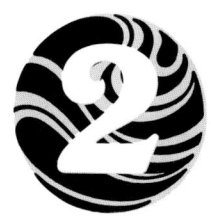

A QUICK DIP INTO THE HISTORY OF BATHING

Getting yourself into hot water usually means big trouble. With the exception of a hapless missionary or two who once upon a time found himself on simmer this expression shouldn't evoke a negative response. People have been getting into hot water since earliest times—and loving every minute of it!

Our planet is made of hot gasses with a cooler crust over it that we call terra firma. But the earth still has residual hot spots welling up all over its surface in the form of active volcanoes, geysers and hot springs. Obviously, a volcano wouldn't be much fun as hot spots go, nor would a steaming geyser, but natural hot springs have always been favorite soaking spots for animals and mankind alike.

The early Romans really knew how to utilize a hot spot. They built enormous stone baths in magnificent mosaic temples, which were the favorite socializing and relaxing centers of Roman society. The baths included such niceties as lounging areas, dressing rooms, drinking wells, and even a spray for intimate showering. Ruins of the elaborate baths and aqueducts built by the Romans still survive in Italy, England, France and West Germany. That some of the ruins and aqueducts are still used today is a tribute to the Roman architectual genius, as well testimony to the universal love of bathing.

The Greeks, also famous for bathing, primarily used the bath as a necessary part of a gymnastic regimen; their baths were often brief, cold and invigorating—*Let's go out there and get 'em, team!* The Turkish baths, utilizing heat and steam, are still very popular all over the world, as are the Finnish and Swedish dry-heat saunas.

Bathing and washing have always had special ritual uses in religion, magic and chivalry, which really transcend cleanliness; for these purposes, bathing was a means of achieving ablution. Moslems and Hindus bathe for ritual purposes, and the Mosaic Code of the Jews requires ritual bathing.

In the medieval monastery, adhering to rules of penance and self-denial, the bath was used strictly for cleansing. Any pleasure derived from the icy water was purely spiritual.

King Henry IV founded the Order of the Bath to teach that cleanliness was indeed next to godliness, but apparently his knights needed little encouragement. They took to bathing like ducks to water, for one woodcut illustration in a thirteenth century manuscript depicted a young knight being offered a bath with young maidens in attendance. Another illustration shows a knight soaking in his wooden tub while a pretty young lady is showering him with rose petals. (Perhaps there's a double meaning to the expression, "when knighthood was in flower?") Other woodcuts show a communal tub with a tray of food and drink across it, while another shows musicians playing to a tub full of bathers. In medieval stories of amorous adventures, it was common for two lovers to begin the evening by bathing together. It appears no one was terribly

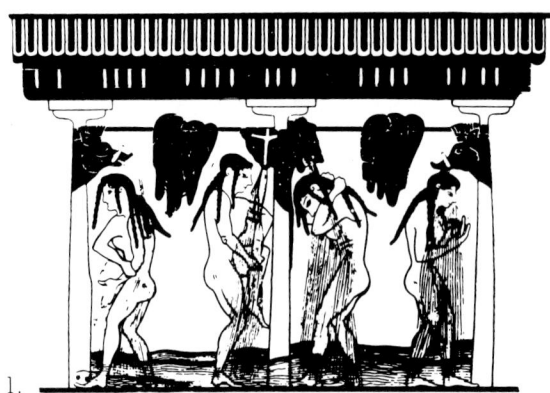
1.

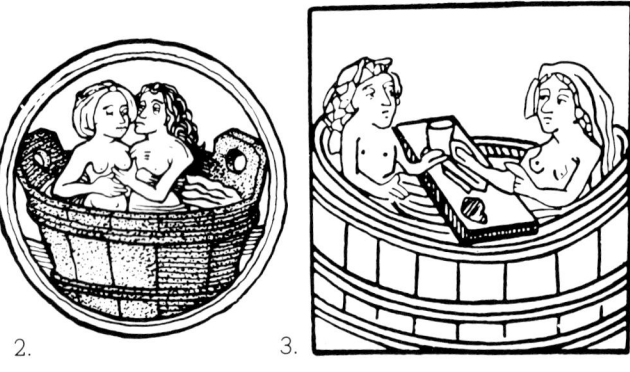
2.

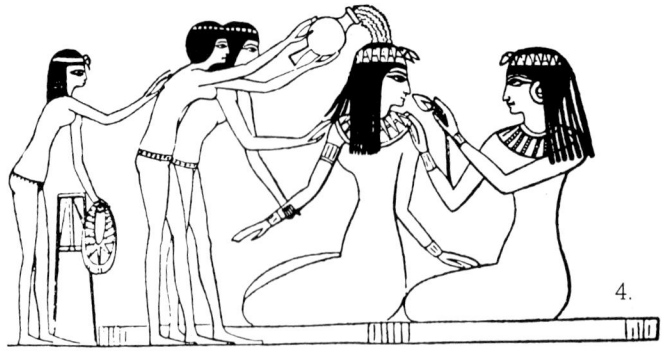
3.

Communal bathing isn't new; some societies were just more advanced in the art than others. 1. Minoan Crete had better facilities than Victorian England. 2 & 3. Bathing has always encouraged enjoying the delights of the flesh. 4. Egyptian tombs show the ancient cleansing rites that were only for the powerful. 5. This sixteenth century woodcut reveals a Turkish woman's bathing costume, and one reason the Crusades were fought. 6. The early European baths, or "stews," fell into disuse because of the fear of disease caused by the Plague. 7. The "Turkish" bath was reintroduced to England during the 1800s. 8. This court jester teasing the ladies was found tooled on a fifteenth century leather casket.

A Quick Dip Into the History of Bathing

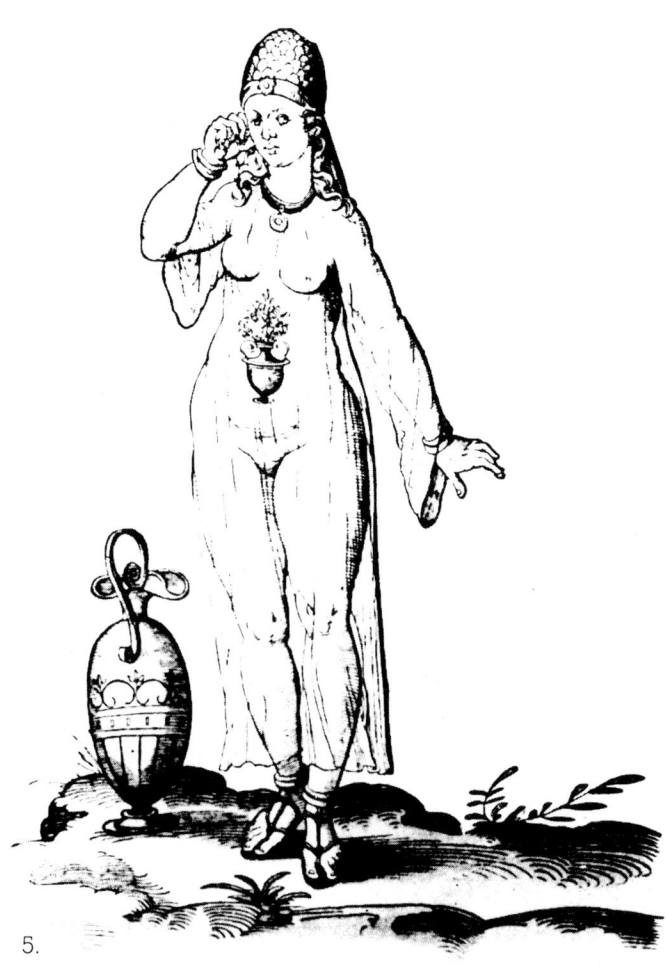

5.

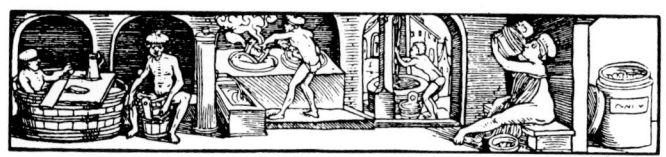

6.

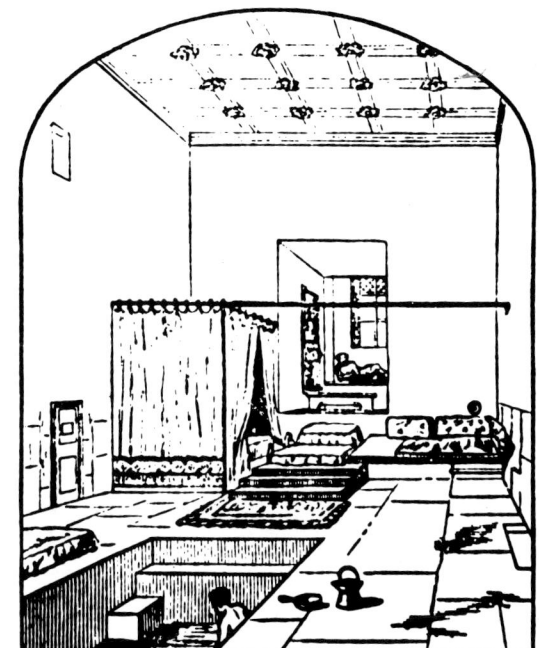

7.

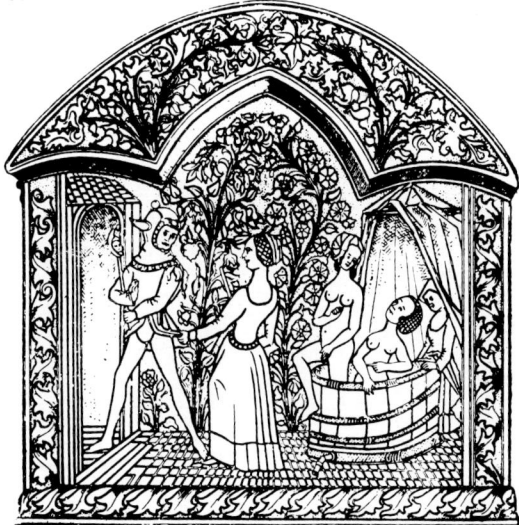

8.

shy about nudity; usually an entire household shared the same sleeping compartment.

Some fastidiously declined to bathe, whether for moral reasons or perhaps simply they never noticed that they smelled bad. King John of England bathed about once a month, it's said, usually in preparation for church festivities; following suit, his subjects presumably bathed less often. Queen Isabella of Spain claimed to have had only two baths in her life!

In the fifteenth century, monks and physicians loudly condemned the public baths as hot beds of vice, sloth and excessive drinking. The Church of England opposed the baths so strongly that Christians began to go dirty as penance for their sins. There were strong laws against bathing in the early American colonies because the Puritans felt bathing encouraged promiscuity because of the nudity involved. Any mention of bathing or bodily functions became shameful and sinful. These attitudes carried over into the Victorian era, where in one early advertisement a bathtub was shown disguised as a couch!

Though bathing has always been a measure of the health and hygiene of a civilization, early illustrations show the interest in the society around the baths. 9. Revelry in the stews in Nuremberg from an etching by Dürer. 10. In Elizabethan England the tubs were filled by water carriers. 11. The bath was central to the amorous tales of knights in the courtly tradition. 12. Here it appears that a monk has been left to attend to the needs of the ladies as they soak under their canopies. 13. The bath was a natural place for intrigue and dramatic turns of events.

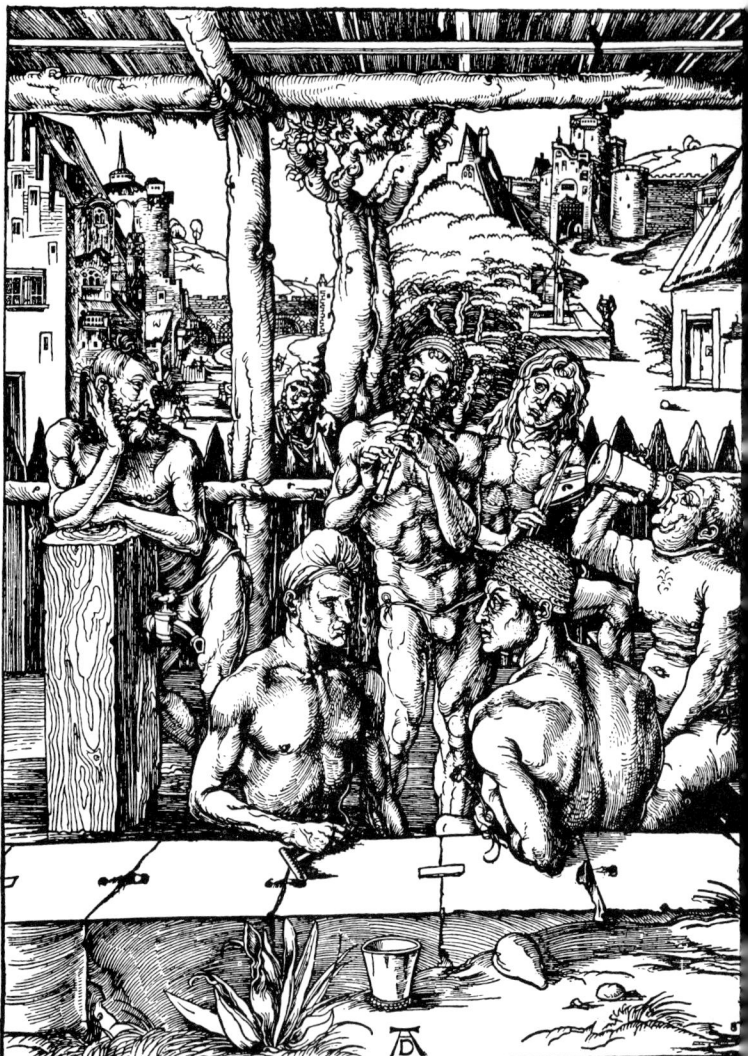

9.

A Quick Dip Into the History of Bathing

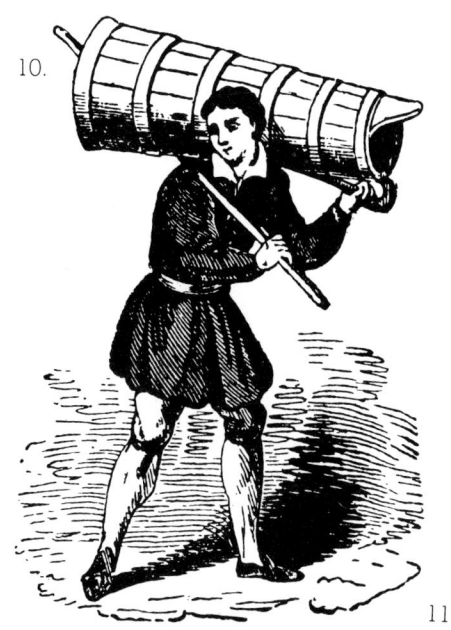

10.

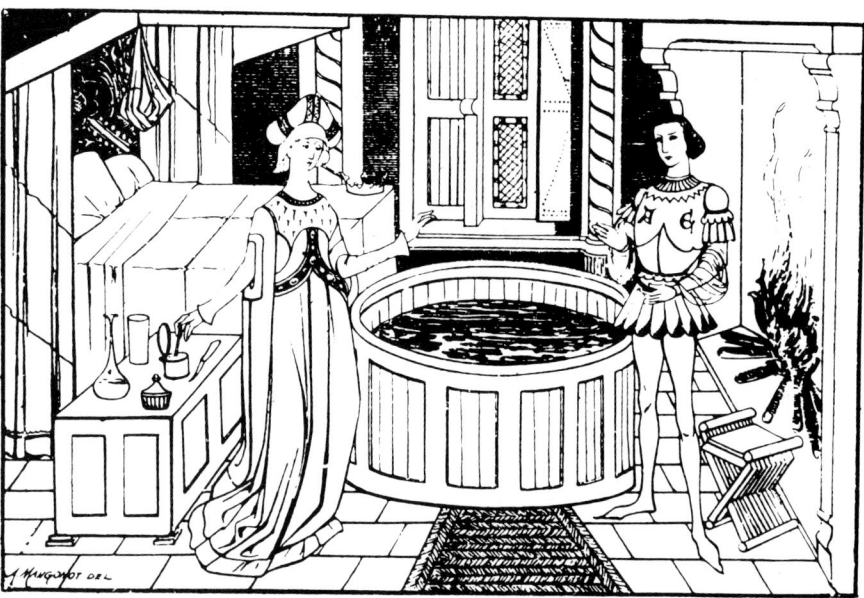

11.

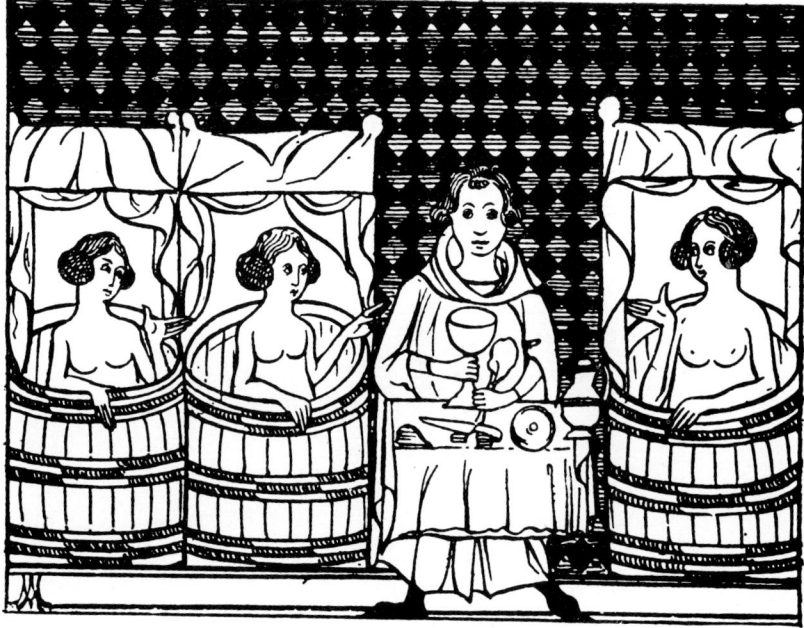

12.

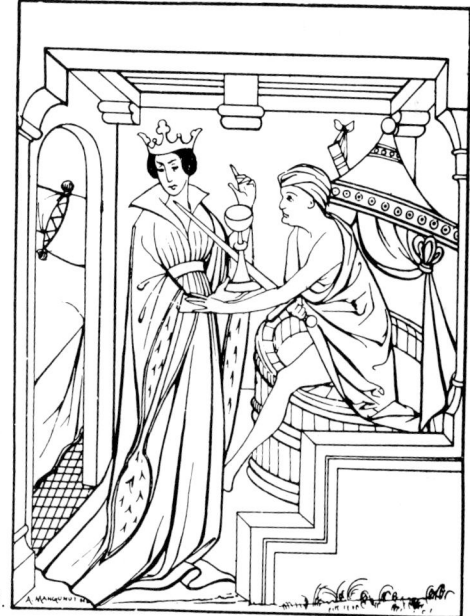

13.

CANNIBAL SOUP

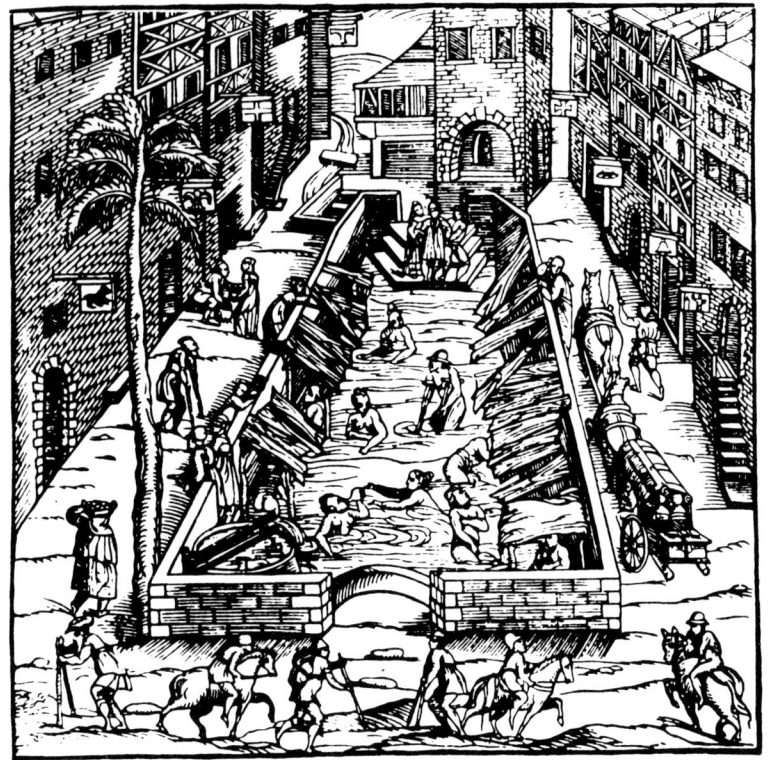

14.

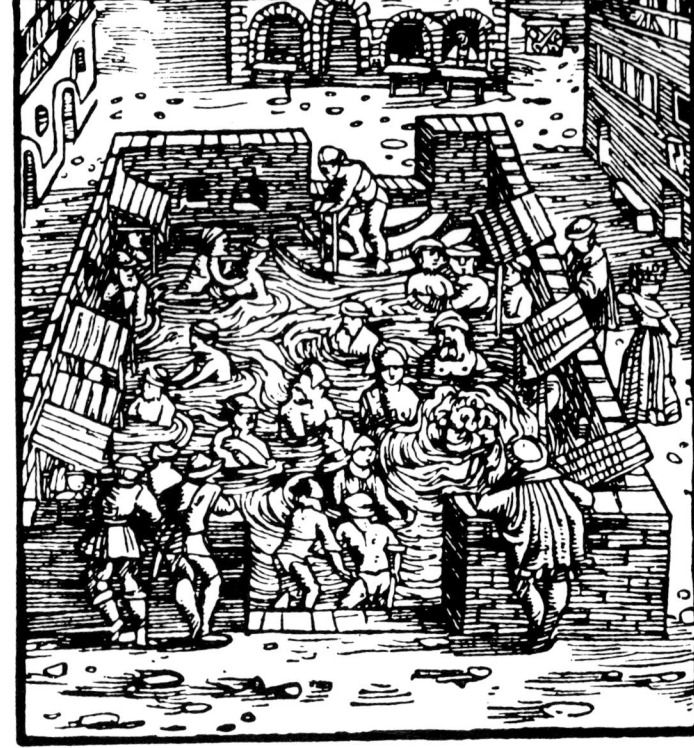

15.

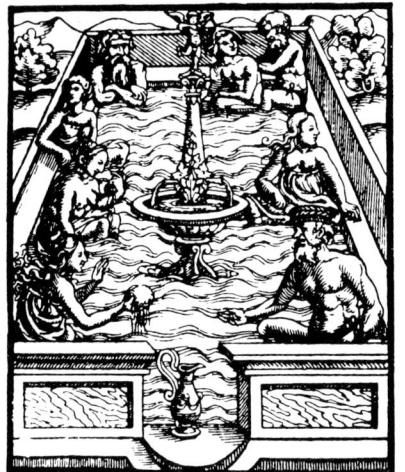

16.

The spa developed in Europe on the models of the Roman and Turkish baths—surrounded by pubs (14-17). 18. A bathtub from King Minos' palace. 19. A half-bath for soaking in the livingroom. 20. A tub made of sheet-metal and shaped like a boot for modesty and warmth.

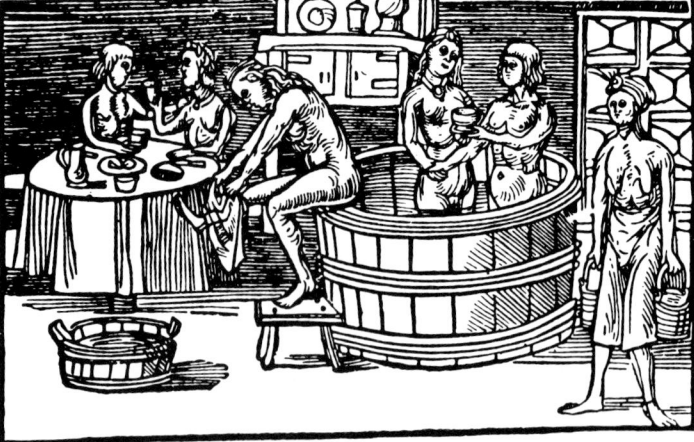

17.

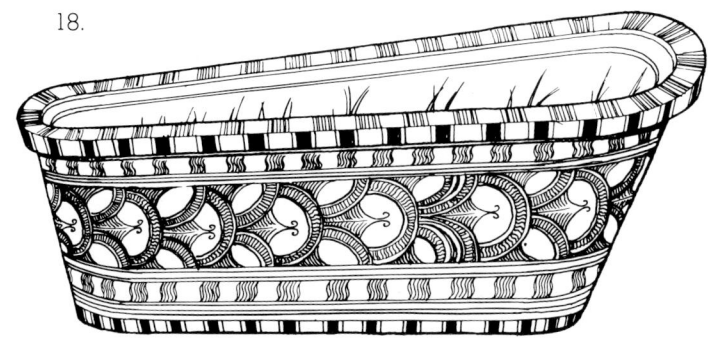

18.

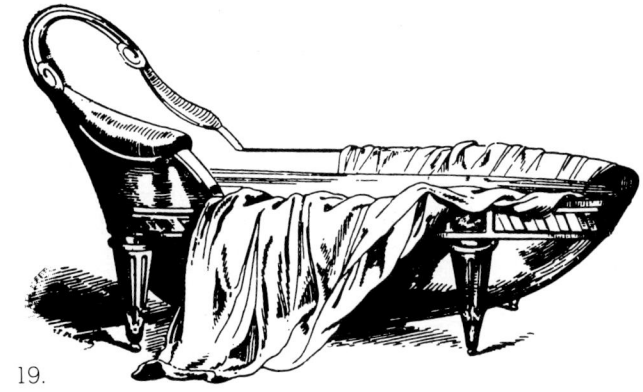

19.

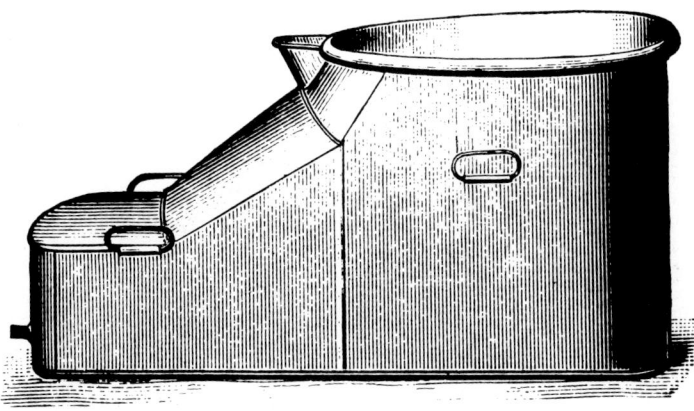

20.

These attitudes have not, of course, gone down the drain. Our modern-day bathing habits reflect our obsession for efficiency and cleanliness—three-minute showers, chrome and porcelain fixtures, bright white uncomfortable bathtubs and commodes—all of which conspire to give our modern bathrooms the charm and beauty of a sterile hospital room. Clean, clean, *clean*! Whatever happened to soaking for relaxation and socialization?

The Japanese have kept their bathing senses and their passion for bathing is proverbial. The Japanese take a hot bath at least once a day, washing off outside the tub, then soaking leisurely in their indoor tub, the *ofuro*. Almost every home has an *ofuro*, and those people who don't, visit the public bath houses. The Japanese enjoy the water hotter than most Westerners, and emerge from the 113°F. water "as red as a boiled octopus." The hot springs which abound in volcano-studded Japan are also extremely popular with these bath-lovers.

Hot springs, wherever found, have always been popular health and resort areas. Among the famous resorts are Bath, England; Baden-Baden, in West Germany; Aix-les-Bains in the French Alps; Saratoga Springs, New York, and the Arkansas Hot Springs. "Taking the baths" was one of the favorite activities of the carriage set of the Gay Nineties. Soon the plush resorts and hotels became known worldwide for their curative benefits. In the late nineteenth century, ailing author Robert Louis Stevenson took his bride to Calistoga Springs, California, for their honeymoon, and then settled in nearby Silverado. He attributed to the thermal springs and warm countryside his regaining his health. Stories abound of miraculous recoveries from illness after bathing or drinking mineral waters, and the popularity of hot springs bathing persists today, although many of the plush resorts of the *belle époque* have lapsed into ruin or been destroyed by fire.

One of the hottest spots on the West Coast since the early sixties has been the baths at the Esalen Institute in Big Sur, California. Here in a relaxing, natural environment many of the current self-awareness techniques were born. From the encounter groups and sensitivity training sessions have emerged such influential figures as Fritz Perls, of the Gestalt therapy; Abraham Maslow, known for his work in humanistic psychology; and Ida Rolf, whose system of deep massage is practiced by many today.

The baths at Esalen are open to the public after midnight on Sunday evenings, and for a minimal fee one can enjoy the flavor of the Roman baths. While not as large or as elaborate as the Roman temples, Esalen offers many large stone tubs which sit under a shelter open on one side to a magnificent view of the waves rushing onto the rocks below. Bathers meditate or practice Esalen massage techniques; the sea breeze slowly cools your heated body. The only negative feature, as with all mineral baths, is the peculiar odor of sulphur, iron, magnesium, and other minerals in the water. This faint odor, reminiscent, frankly, of rotten eggs, is easy to get used to, and is a small price to pay for the re-

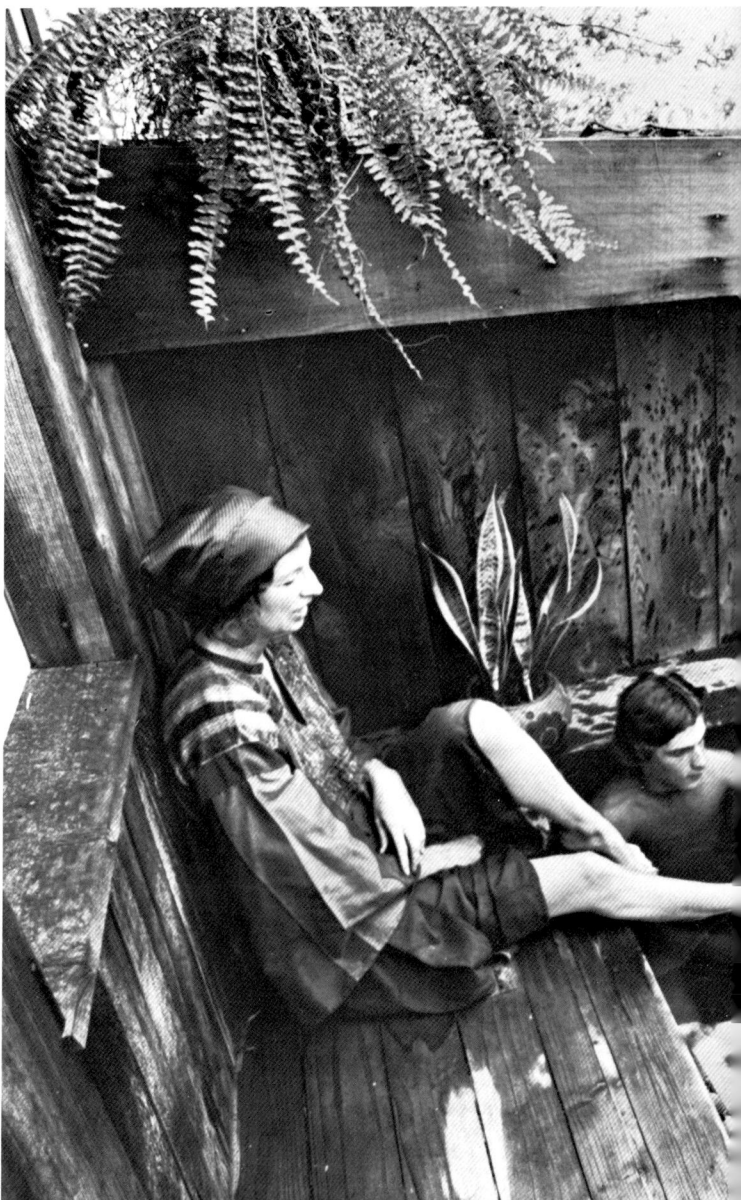

The hot tub provides a place for the modern-day family to sit together surrounded by nature and to peacefully talk.

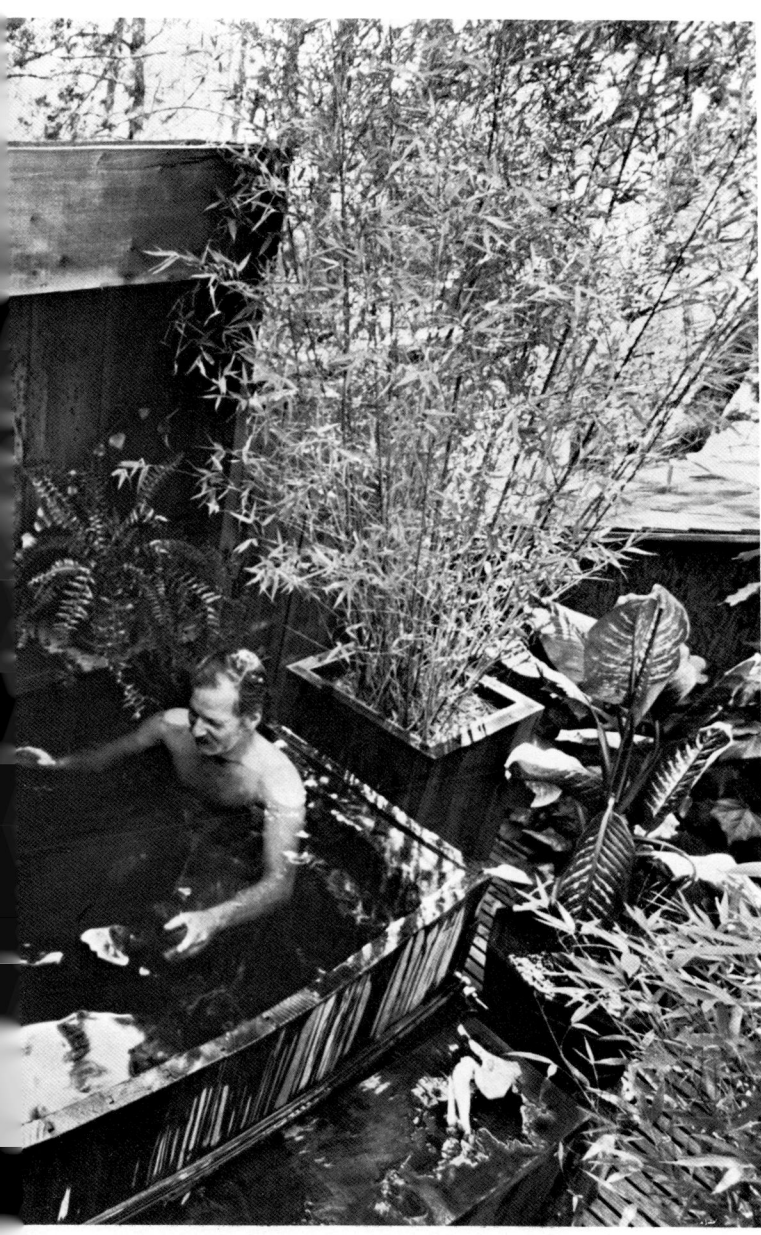

wards of a hot bath among a company of friendly bathers.

Now, thanks to an innovative soaking tub devised by some Santa Barbara war veterans with warm memories of the Japanese *ofuros,* we can all enjoy the luxury of the Roman baths; the sensual pleasures of the medieval baths; the family and communal socializing of the Japanese baths; and the creative value of natural hot springs bathing. It is here—the redwood hot tub!

This simple tub, old as the two-thousand-year-old redwoods themselves, has been modernized with the addition of filters, heaters and therapy jets. It has revolutionized today's bathing habits. The spic-and-span spa made of tile and coping like a swimming pool can't begin to compete with the soft, sensual appeal of natural redwood next to your body. And, if you surround the tub with trees, bamboo or hanging plants, your redwood tub will *feel* as much at home and contented as you do!

Recently, scientists and oceanographers discovered a volcanic hot spot in the bottom of the Pacific Ocean. Normal bottom water in the area of the Galapagos Rift Zone is a cool 35°F., but among the lava vents and geysers of the rift zone, the temperature measures a warm 61°F. Startled scientists on this straight-laced research project reported that they saw fish swimming around in the warm water with big smiles on their faces!

Today, thousands of happy hot-tub owners are discovering the pure joy of "getting into hot water." Birds do it. We do it. Even fishes in the sea do it. Communal bathing is here again, and are we ever glad. Fifty million bathers can't be wrong! *C'mon in, the water's fine!*

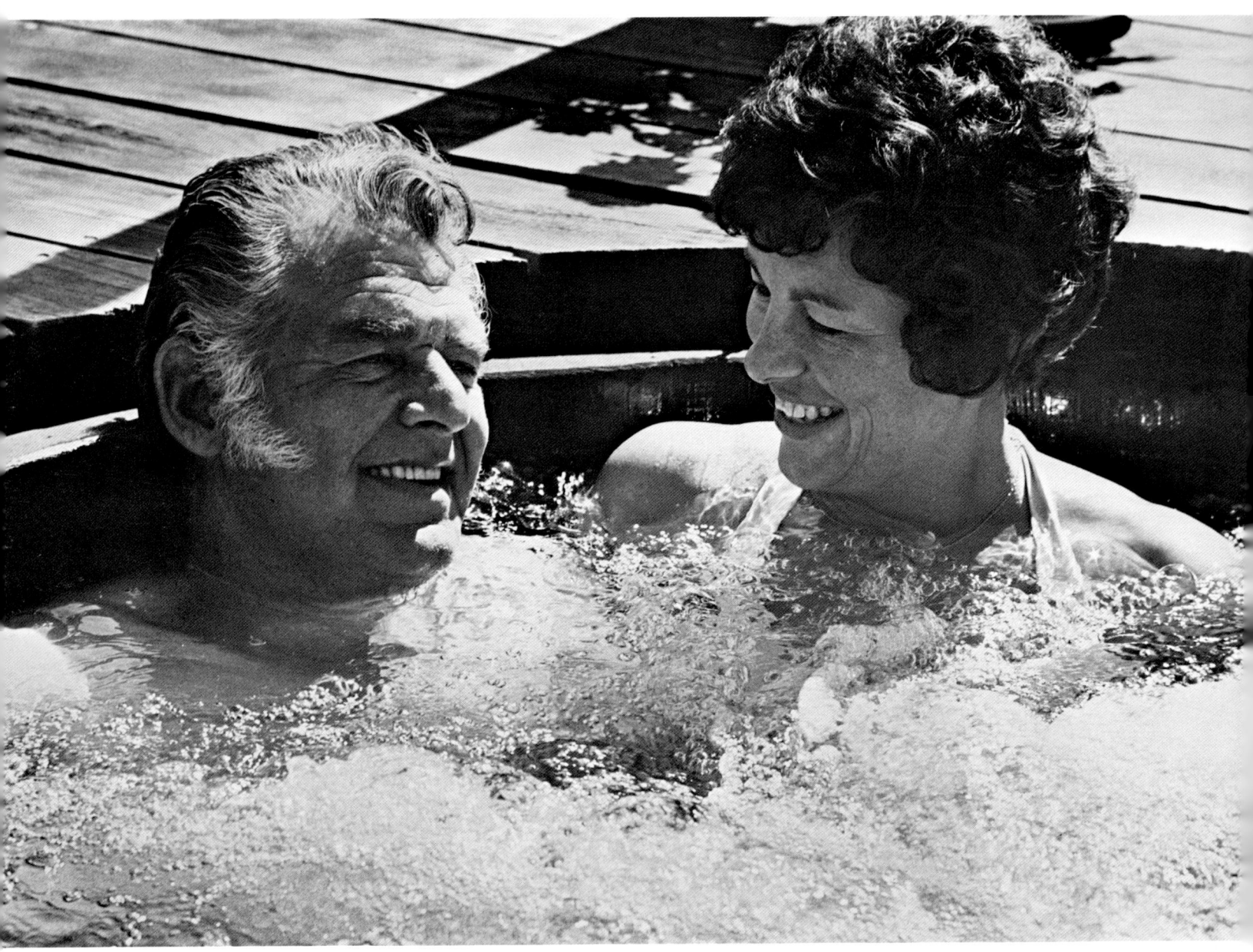

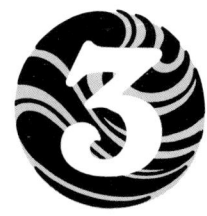

THE RENAISSANCE OF THE HOT TUB

The emergence of the hot-tub phenomenon was brought about by a few imaginative and adventurous souls in Santa Barbara, California, who made their first hot tubs out of used water tanks and wine vats. Cleaned, repaired and modified, these tubs, equipped with salvaged pumps and heaters, were transformed into steaming tubs ready to accommodate the happy people who'd made them. As the demand for this new product grew, the supply of ready-made vats dwindled. A small company was formed and new tubs were custom-built rather than scavenged from old tanks. Thus, the art of cooperage was reborn—a craft that had all but been forgotten. Like a mythical phoenix, cooperage was reborn just as it was almost completely destroyed by modern assembly lines and steel barrels. May the hot tub be as immortal!

The revival of enthusiasm over the modern-day hot tub spread rapidly throughout California and is washing across the nation. Hot-tub converts have a special treat awaiting them, for there is nothing more satisfying than lingering in a steaming barrel of water while the world rushes madly by. The tubber with a snowy winter has his own special hot tub treat—snow. Crisp, cold, drifting snow accentuates the warmth of a tub filled with 106°F. water. Conversely, the cold snow seems to radiate an invitation to cool off by running or rolling in its icy white softness: the ultimate "sauna" experience.

A hot tub will cost more than a new color TV, but it will also offer you much, much more. A hot tub isn't like a TV set, which sits bulkily in the corner waiting for you to turn it on and watch it passively. Your hot tub will beckon you, invite and cajole you. It's warm and seems alive. Unlike the TV, it will turn *you* on. In spite of yourself, you will gravitate toward it, not simply because it feels so good, but because like bodies do attract, and your body is made up of three-quarters water. You will find that the hot tub's soothing warmth will affect your general well-being and outlook on life for the better. We can't promise that you'll become rich or famous, but you will become more *aware* of yourself. It's been said, "Clothes make the man." But what's left after the clothes are gone? Would your friends still like you on this natural basis—face to face, with no facades? Will you?

We found ourselves facing the naked truth with our friends soon after we bought our tub. We invited two couples, longtime friends, to visit and to share the hot tub with us one weekend. One couple was pleased and filled with anticipation at the prospect of *au naturel* communal bathing, but as the relaxed and pleasant evening drew on and the time of the great descent into the hot tub approached, this same couple became very quiet and withdrawn. They declined the group experience and waited until the rest of us got out before they went in. We don't know what went through their minds that night, but when they dressed and left they took our ten-year friendship out the door with them. We can only assume that they weren't quite as ready for nude bathing as they claimed.

Our culture tends to equate nudity with sex, and is really quite fearful of the sight of the naked body—one of the most natural sights in the world. Since we have had our tub, we have seen everything from six-month-old to sixty-year-old bodies. Amazing as it sounds, every single one was beautiful. Even those who look plump in street clothes appeared as natural and graceful as a Reubens nude. We also have seen our share of bathing suits in the tub, as some of our family and friends feel more comfortable that way. We make too much of the vogue and trend of thinness. People are people,

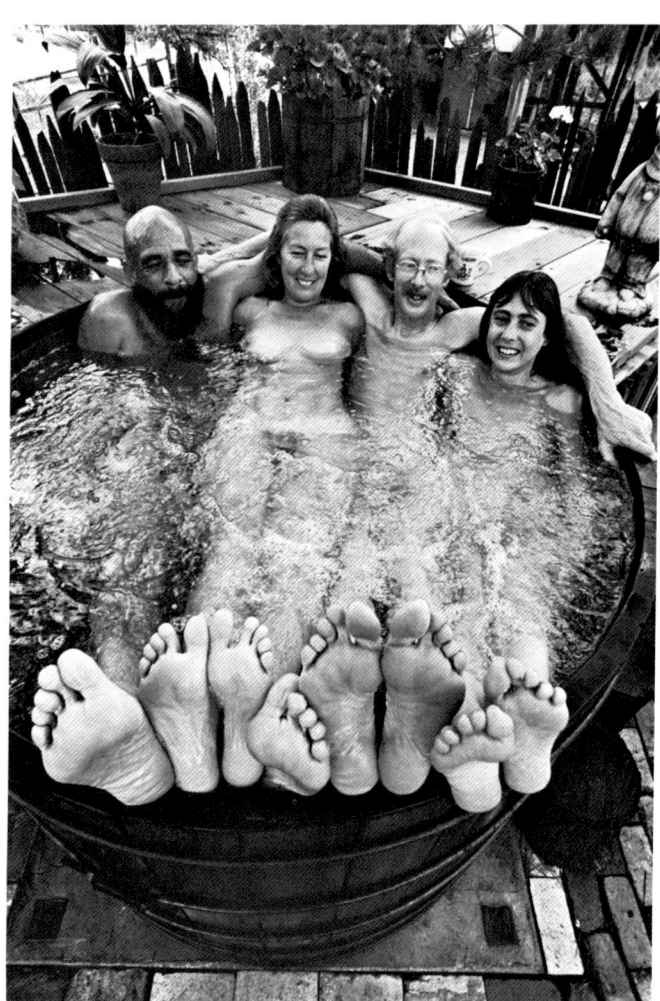

Eight feet in a five-foot tub.

and they come in all shapes and sizes. It's been said that the heart and mind are the only truly erogenous zones. So, try suitless tubbing at least once if you feel comfortable—you may be glad you did.

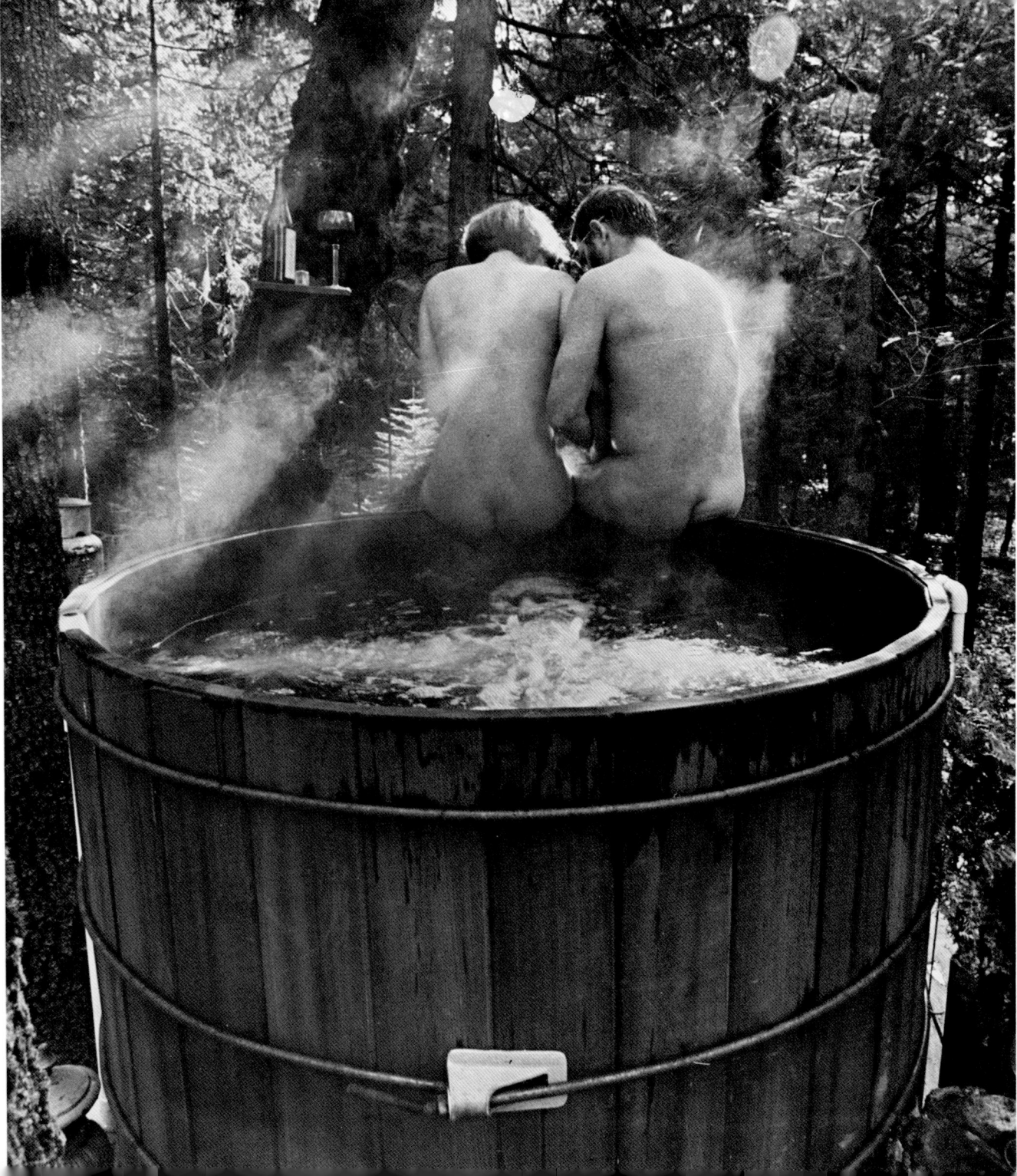

A HOT TUB MAY CHANGE YOUR LIFE

Swimming-pool prices are soaring to astronomical prices only within the reach of an Arab oil sheik or the president of IBM. The hot tub is all the more refreshing for its small price tag. A hot tub is within the reach of practically everyone's budget—it's simply a matter of priorities. Once the initial cost has been laid out, it will cost you no more than the price of running your hot-water heater (approximately 15¢ a day). How else can you indulge yourself so luxuriously for a few cents a day? And at home? Your hot tub will become the hub of your social life. Forget those big entertainment tabs for dinner and a nightclub. Just invite your friends over for a delicious dinner, indulge in your favorite mood-enhancer, and climb into your hot tub. Return to the simple pleasures and take life a little more easily. Your hot tub is designed to help you make this change.

If you're single, there's no better way to get truly acquainted wth a new friend. Now, we don't mean just taking your clothes off—people have been doing that for years without any help from a hot tub. What we do mean is meeting on a one-to-one basis, aided by communion with the powers of nature. The hot tub is a sure-fire exercise in "getting-to-know-you." Try playing one of the games you'll find in Chapter Four, or just hold hands and let the womb with the view overwhelm you. In the softly rocking warm water, you can't help but speak from the heart. There is no need for facades or pretenses. Let your true self bubble up to the surface. Whoever you are it will really be *you*.

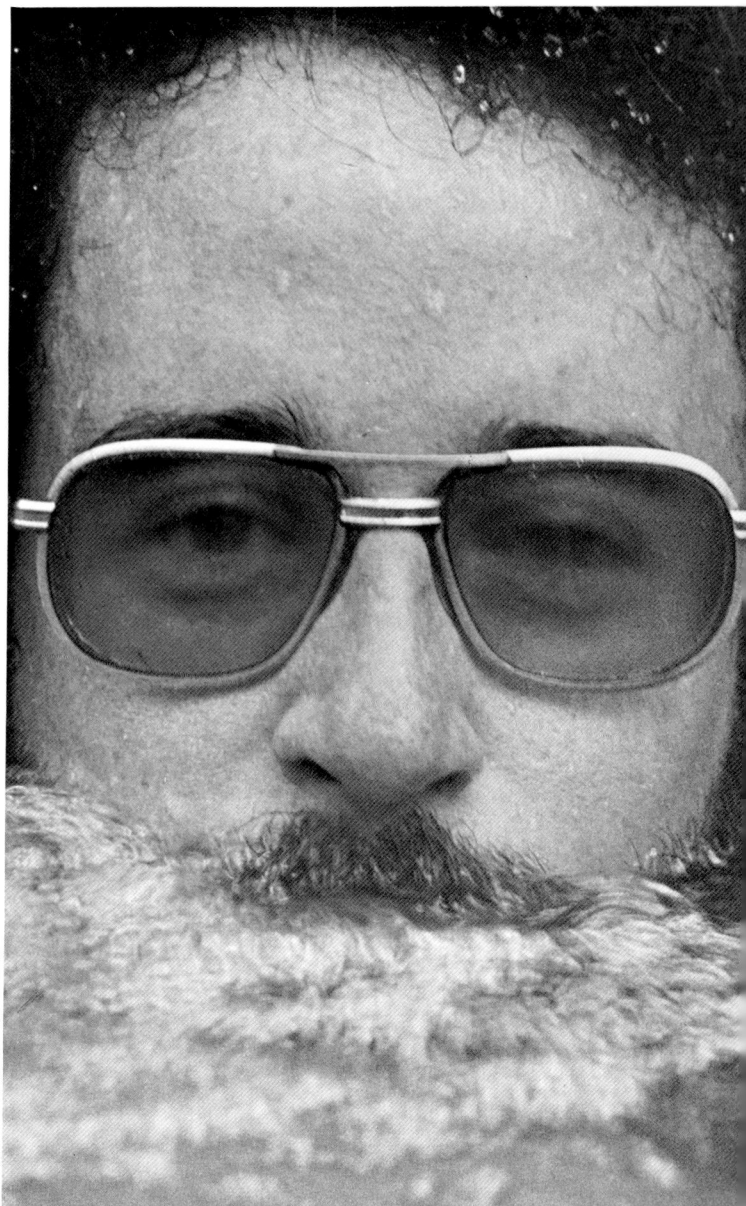

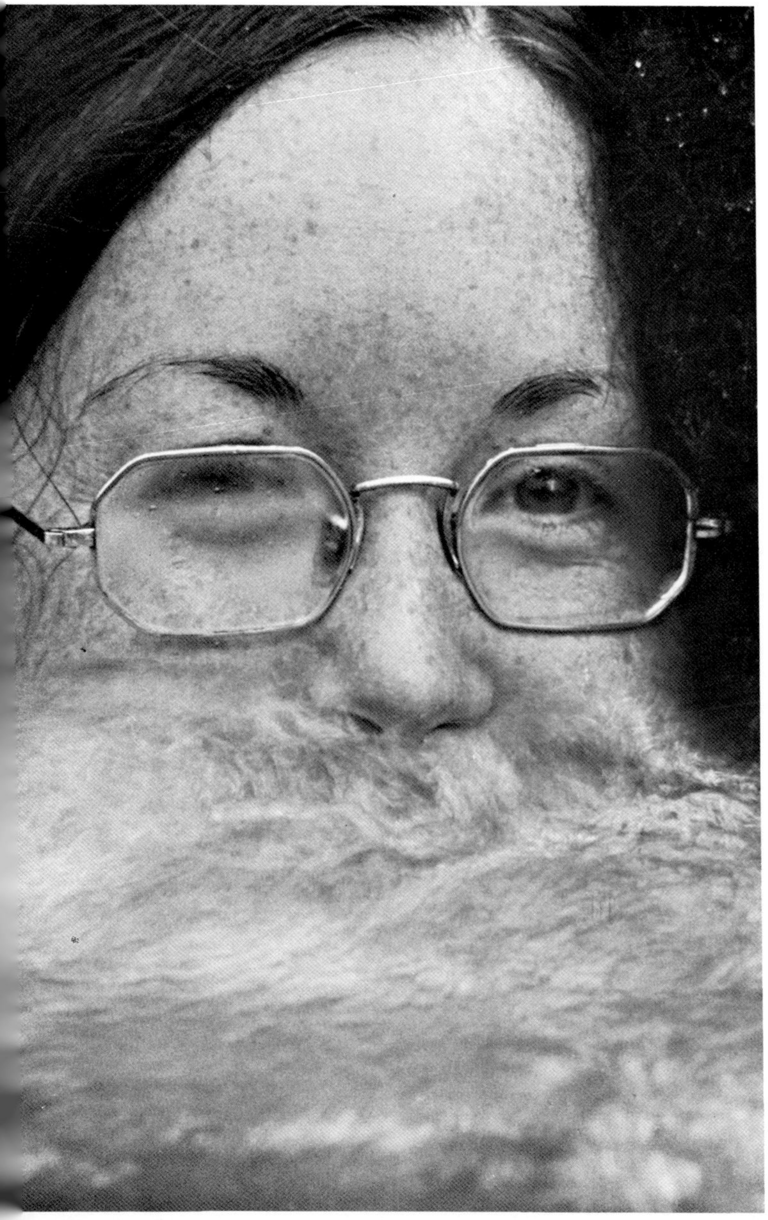

The Renaissance of the Hot Tub

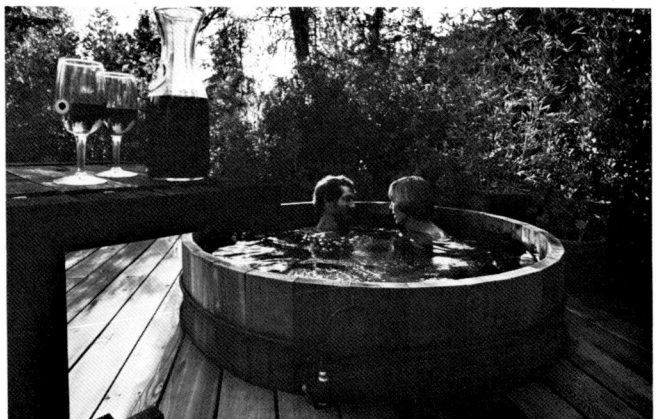

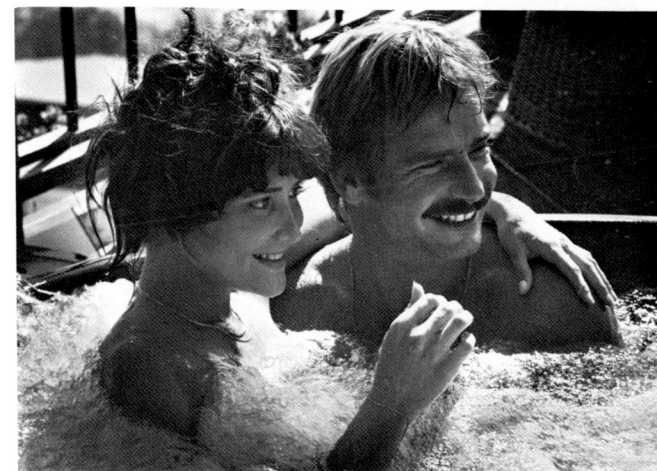

Tubbing à deux.

CANNIBAL SOUP

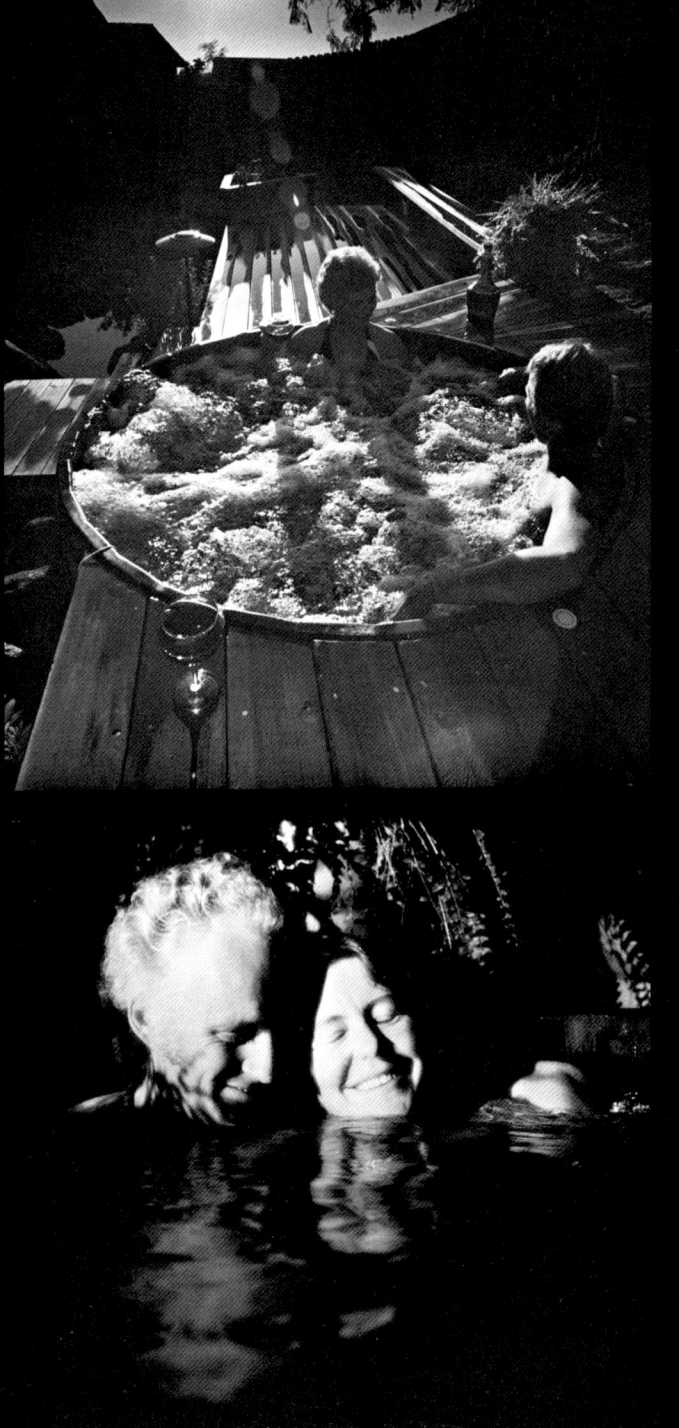

If you're married, you now have a chance to do something very special together: to experience a coupling of minds, rather than bodies. How long has it been since you *really* talked to each other? If you're like most people, you've been so busy working, earning a living; working, raising a family; working, coping with more mundane duties; that sometimes even sex gets relegated to last place. One woman told us, "Every couple needs time to communicate. The only time I see my husband without the kids, TV or with a newspaper in front of his face, is in the hot tub. I can't tell you how much that tub has helped our marriage."

Why not take a half hour each night away from the TV and enjoy a romantic interlude surrounded by millions of shimmering bubbles. You'll discover a renewed closeness and friendship with your mate. For some reason, it is practically impossible to argue in a hot tub. Your petty grievances and irritations seem to slip away as soon as you ease into your sensuous new environment. You two take it from there!

Experience the special kinds of communication that are possible in the intimacy of your hot tub.

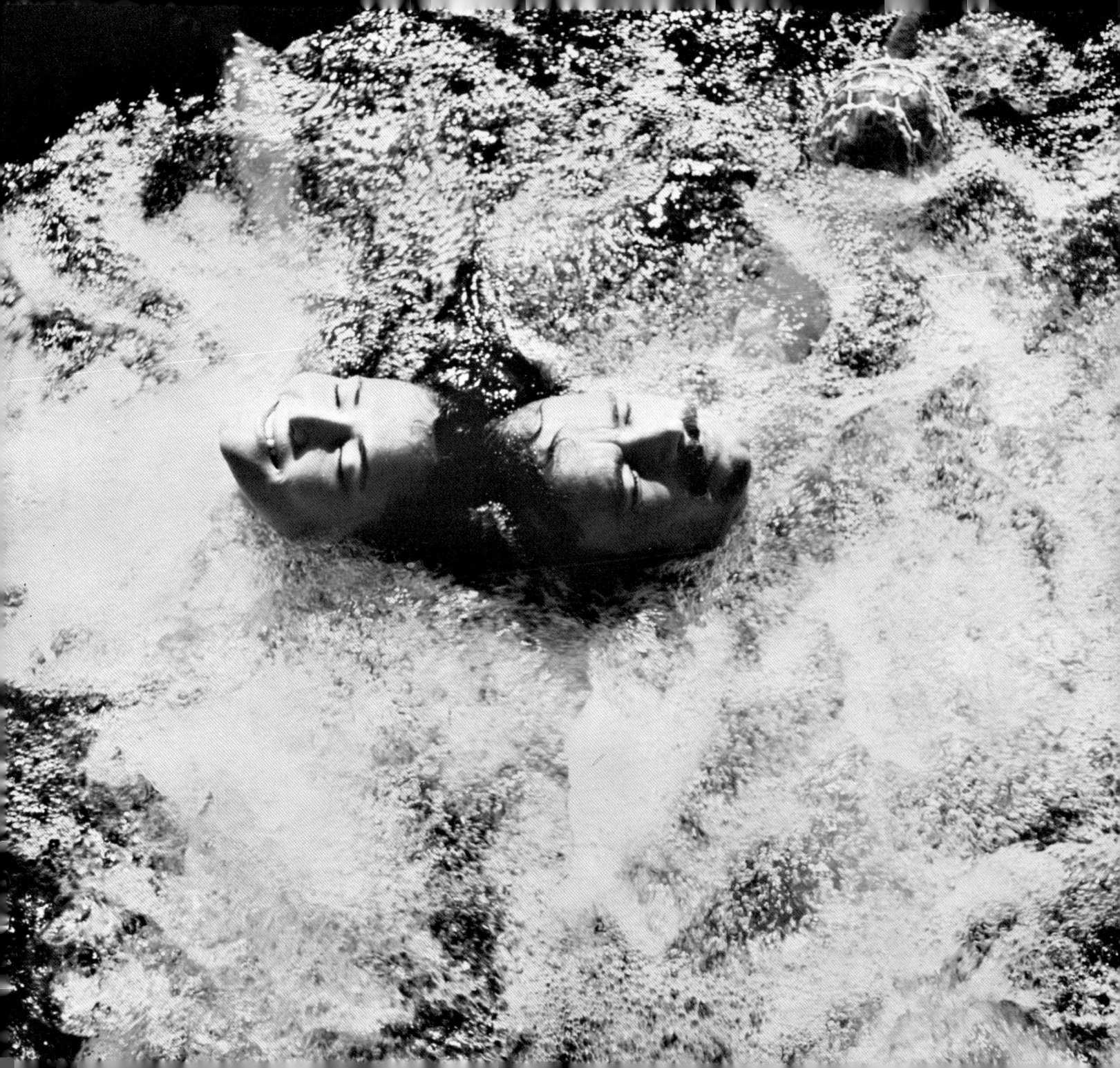

FOR ADULTS ONLY?

We've talked a lot about adult tubbing, now let's discuss children and the hot tub. Many small children fear water, and the sight of a sprawling swimming pool ready to swallow them up forever doesn't help at all. Most of the tiny tots who've seen our wooden keg can't wait to be invited in. Since it doesn't look much bigger than a bathtub, it holds little fear for them. They can stand on a bench inside the tub, grab onto the edges and splash around, or bounce up and down on the bottom of our four-foot tub. The sides of the tub are always within easy reach, so they quickly abandon all fear and splash happily in their small swimming pool. (We usually turn the thermostat down to 102° to 104° F. as children don't seem to like it as hot as adults do.)

Once your child learns how much fun the hot tub is, he may finally consent to those swimming lessons you've been touting. Which brings us to one final point: never leave a child in the vicinity of water without proper supervision. So, join them in the water, or relax on a chaise lounge on the deck—but keep them always under a watchful eye. And, of course, never leave the tub uncovered by the solar blanket or redwood lid when you are to be away for a long time.

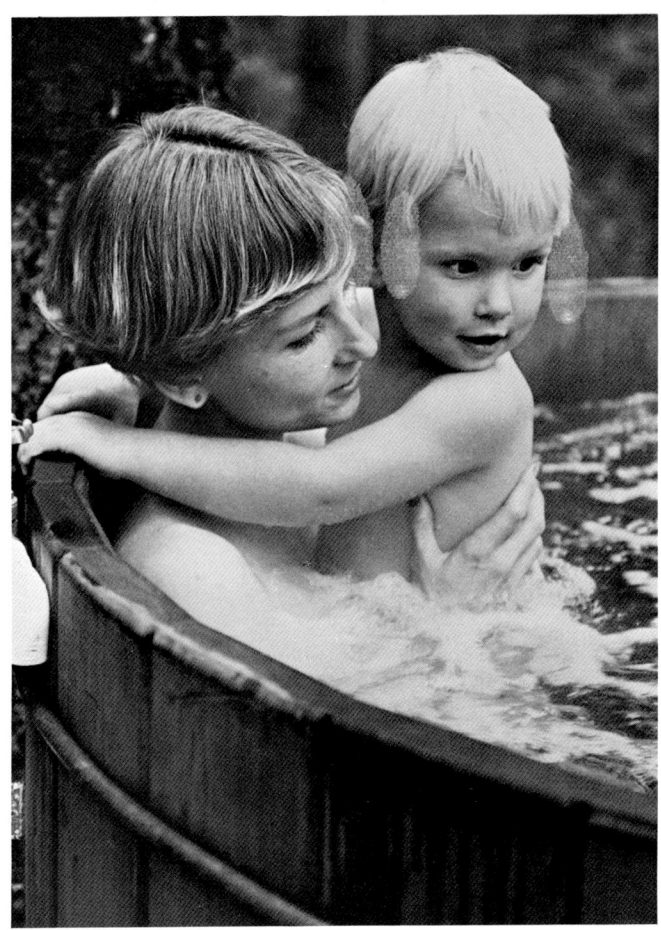

Tubbing with mom or dad adds an extra measure of safety to the water play. Join in your child's enjoyment by bringing his favorite floating toys in with you.

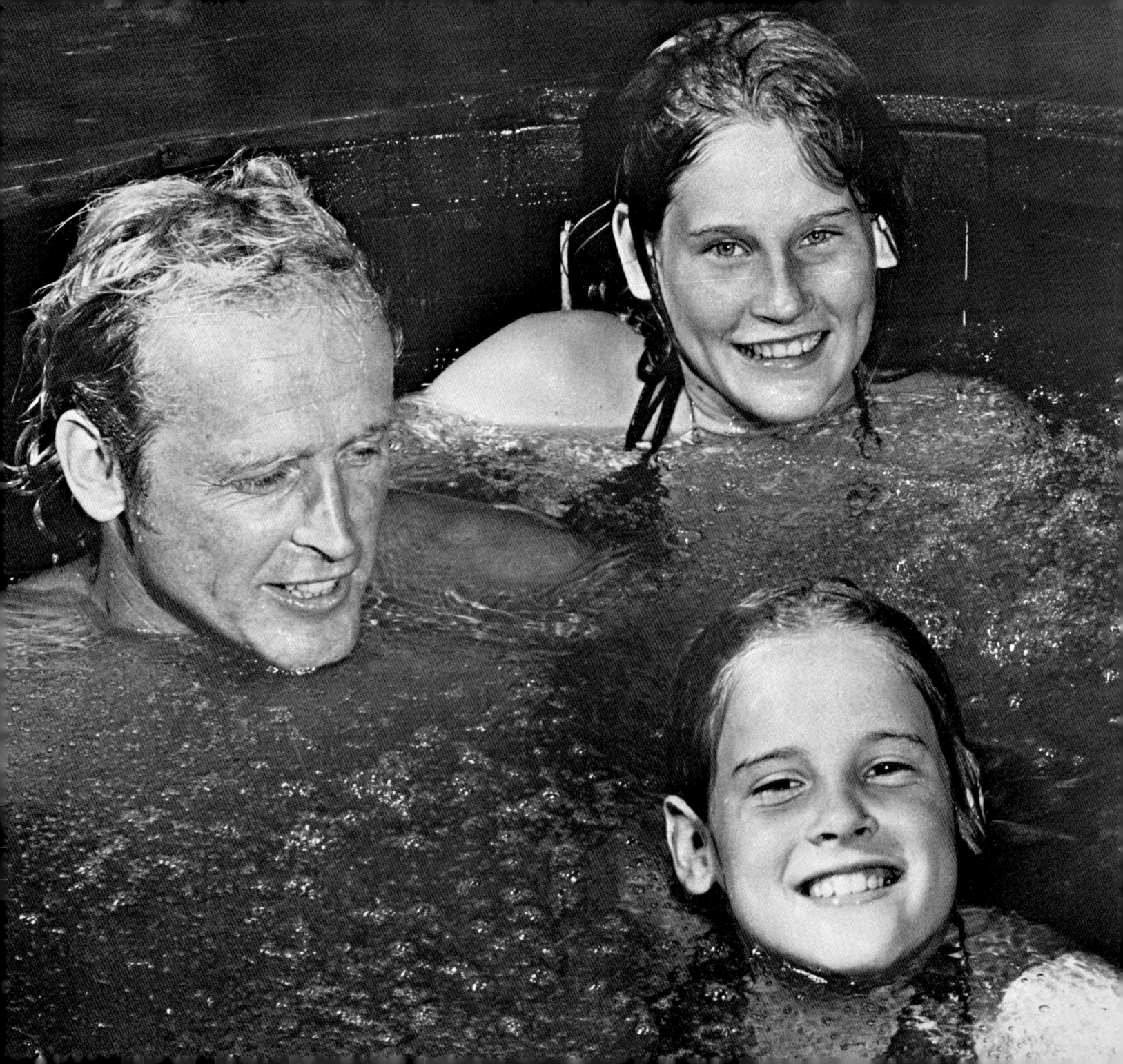

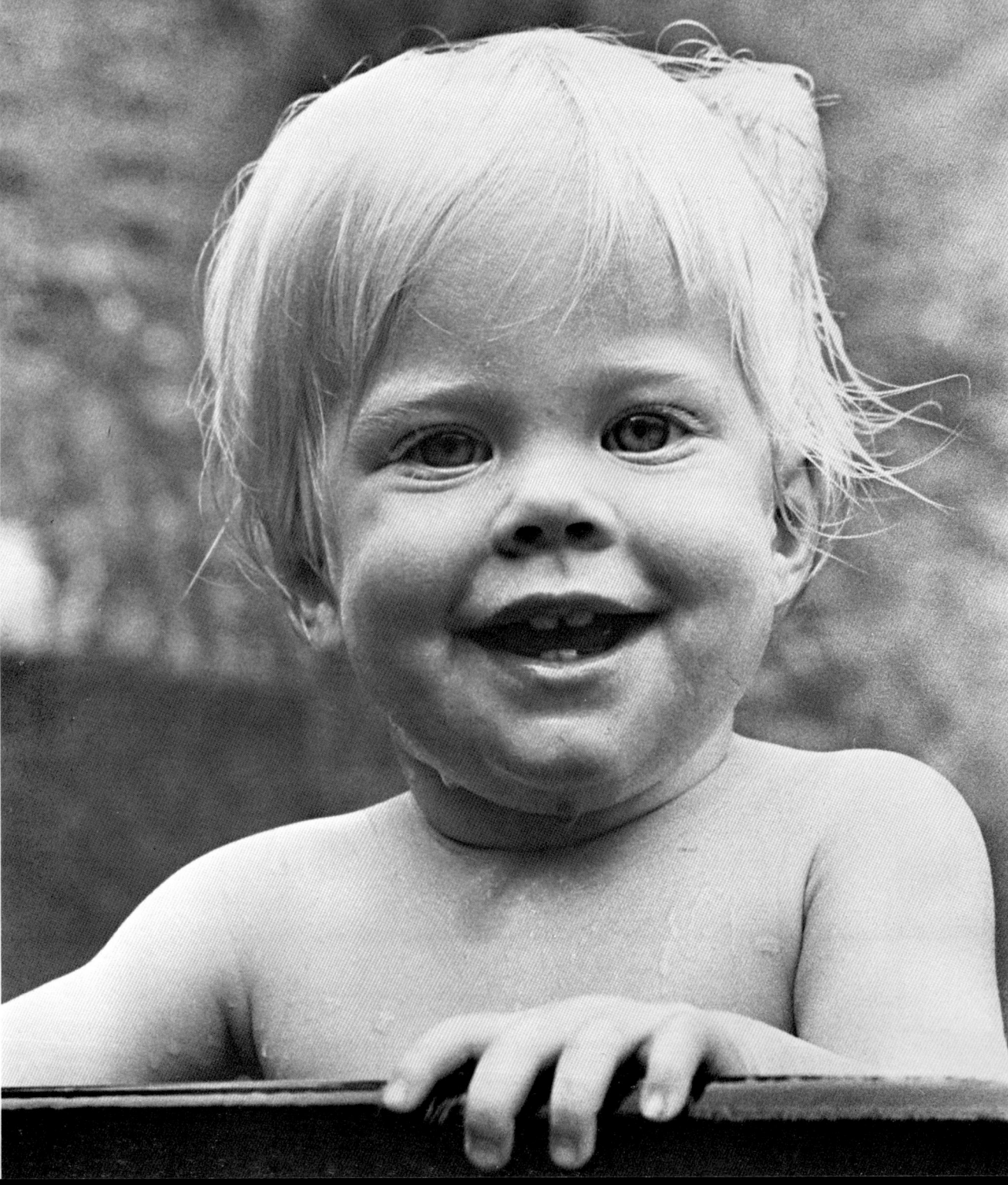

This water baby delights in hot tub play. She fearlessly jumps into the big tub over and over again, each time emerging full of giggles and ready for another splash.

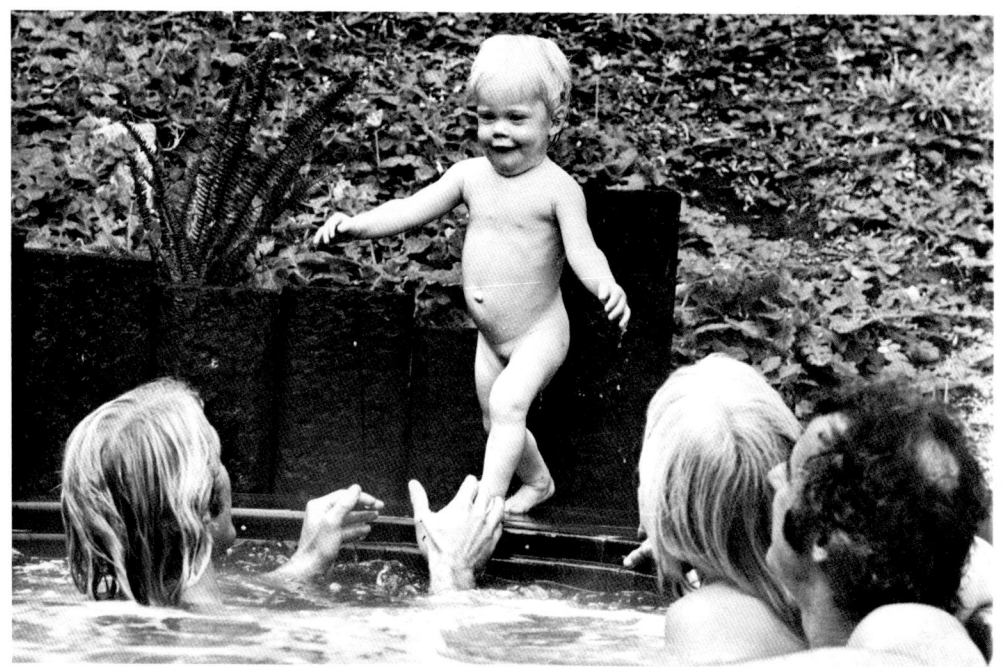

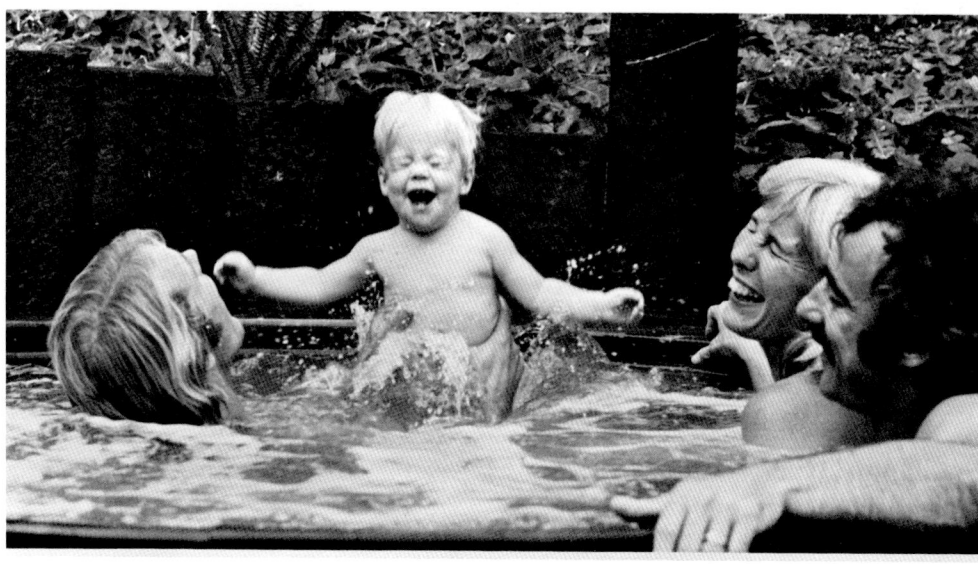

A TUB FOR ALL SEASONS

Another wonderful feature of your hot tub is its dual personality. It can become a "cold tub" in minutes. Just because it's summer and the humidity soars, don't feel your tub is too hot to use. Just turn the thermostat down and run a hose full of cold water into it until your tub is cool. Then climb in and refresh your wilted body in the cold tub while you count your blessings. The kids, too, will be a lot less cranky on those hot summer days if they have a place to take a quick cool dip.

We've already discussed how the hot tub has no regard for snow or heat. So, now to *our* favorite type of weather—rain! No, we're not crazy—rain is always a big cause for celebration around our house. At the first patter of raindrops on our roof, we scramble for the hot tub, where we lay back in the hot steamy water while hundreds of cool raindrops pelt our skin. We turn our faces heavenward and revel in nature's cleansing rite; it's akin to being born again.

Along with the purification of our souls, we delight in the *naughtiness* of staying out in the rain. How many times were we told as children, "Don't get wet—you'll catch your death!" We were shoved into raincoats, bundled into galoshes, scolded if we splashed in an inviting mud puddle, and then hustled off to bed to ward off any chill. Now, grown up and *free*, we can stay out in the rain if we want! We can't catch cold—we're neck-deep in hot water. We don't need coats and hats to keep the water off, 'cause we're already wet! So we can tarry in the storm, tasting the water and reveling in the raindrops dripping on our heads. Then, with a good

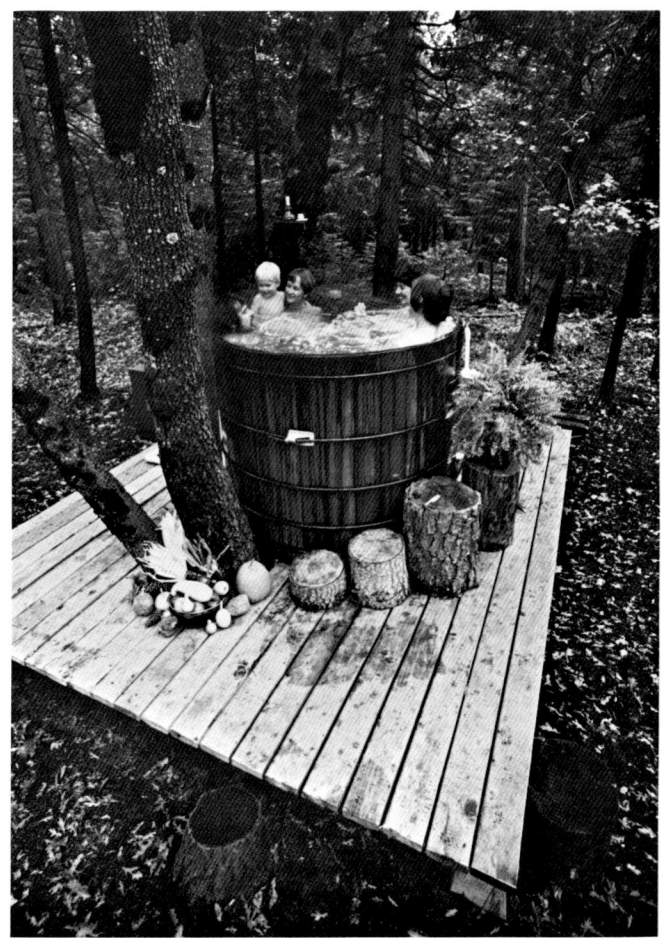

toweling and a warm bathrobe to snuggle into . . . what bliss! Read on, you have only just begun to discover what a hot tub can do for you.

A steaming hot tub is a delightful spot to watch the autumn leaves change color—or to take shelter on a winter day.

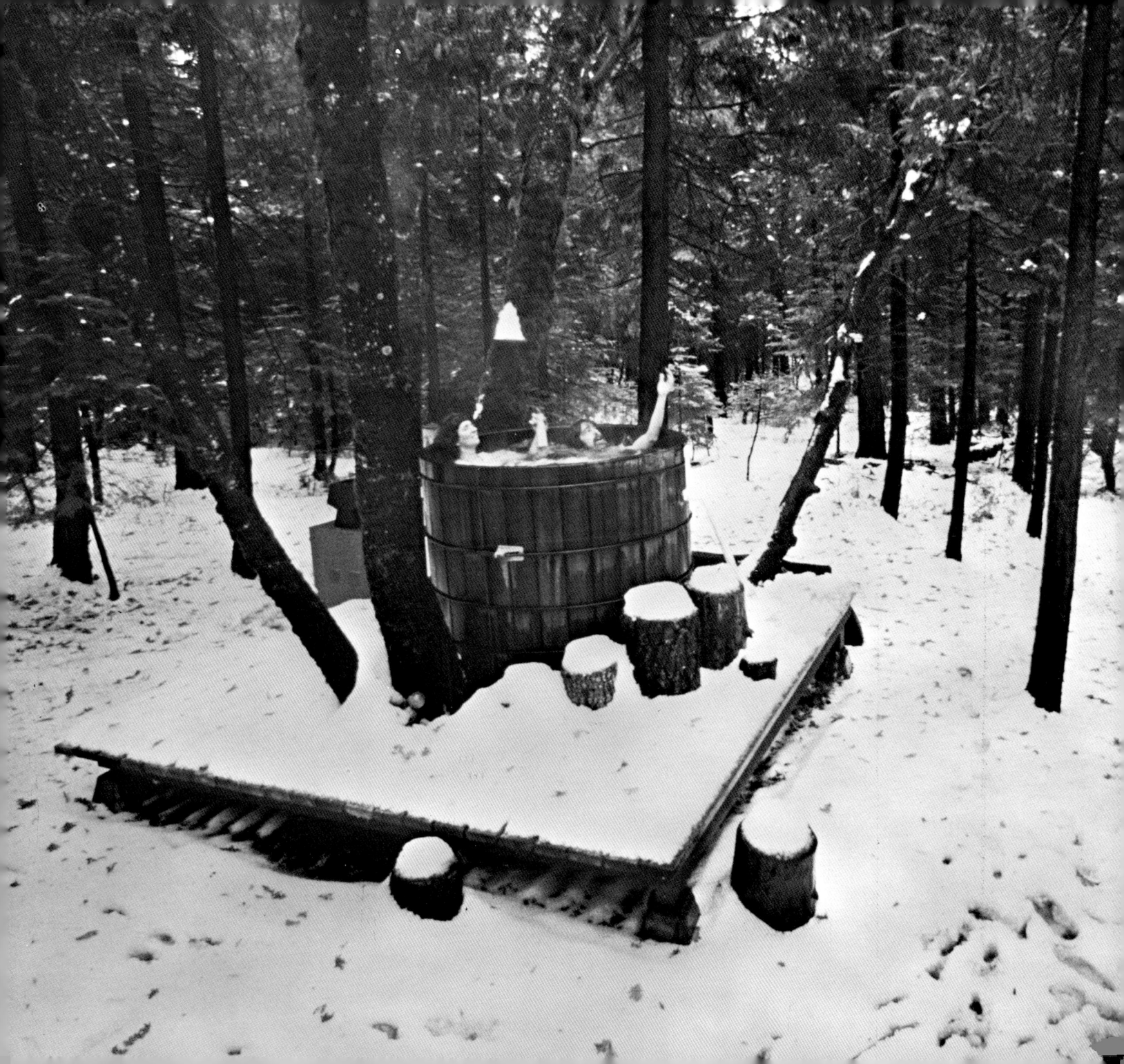

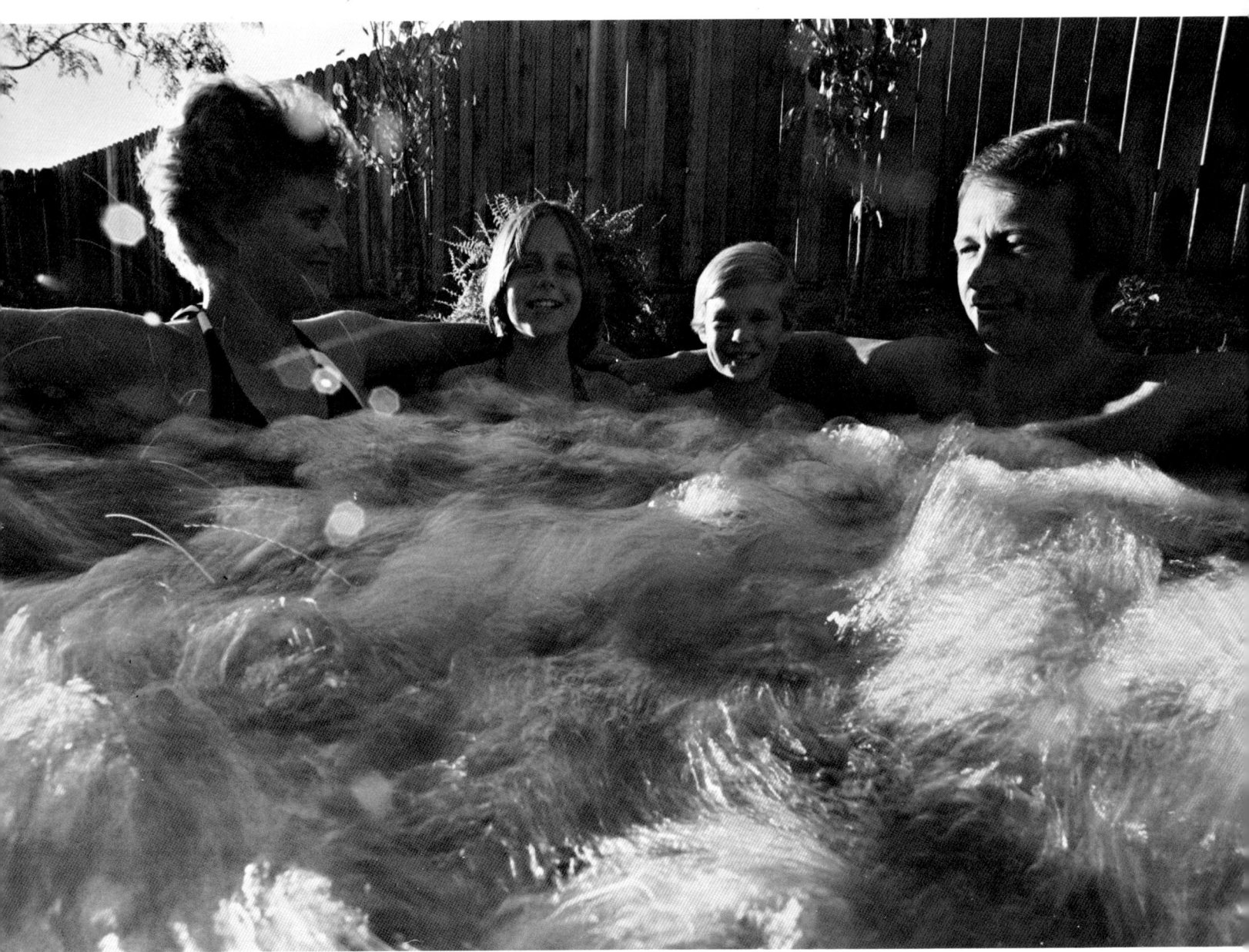

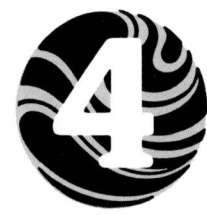

HOT TUB MYTHS AND FANTASIES

ON BEING A GOOD HOT TUB HOST

If you are one of those free spirits who feels totally at ease frolicking on a nude beach, fine. If you normally shed your clothing in the living room and turn floodlights on your hot tub, more power to you. But let's face it—we don't all feel like Mr. Universe or the *Playboy* centerfold, so please be considerate of your guests and their individual modesties. This applies especially to newcomers. Allow them time to shed their inhibitions and their clothes according to their own temperaments. Most people are adventurous at heart and believe in the adage, "When in Rome, do as the Romans do," but give them the option of covering up or baring all! Hand them a large beach towel, or an extra bathrobe before they go off to change, and let them make up their own minds about what they want to wear.

Some people may simply feel more comfortable in a bathing suit, especially if the tub is used during the daylight hours without modesty of moonlight—so let them. Besides, the prospect of parading out to the hot tub in front of God and Everybody Else is tantamount to facing a firing squad for some people. Be a good host or hostess; give your guests a break. You've no doubt extolled the virtues and benefits of *au naturel* tubbing already, and since relaxation and well-being are the purpose of the hot tub experience, why spoil it by insisting upon a certain mode of dress—or undress? Once your newcomer experiences the sensuous pleasure of hot water lapping at his bare skin, his inhibitions may well disappear anyway.

The happy family on the left enjoys extra hydromassage activity, thanks to a newly devised bubble ring unit placed in the bottom of their tub.

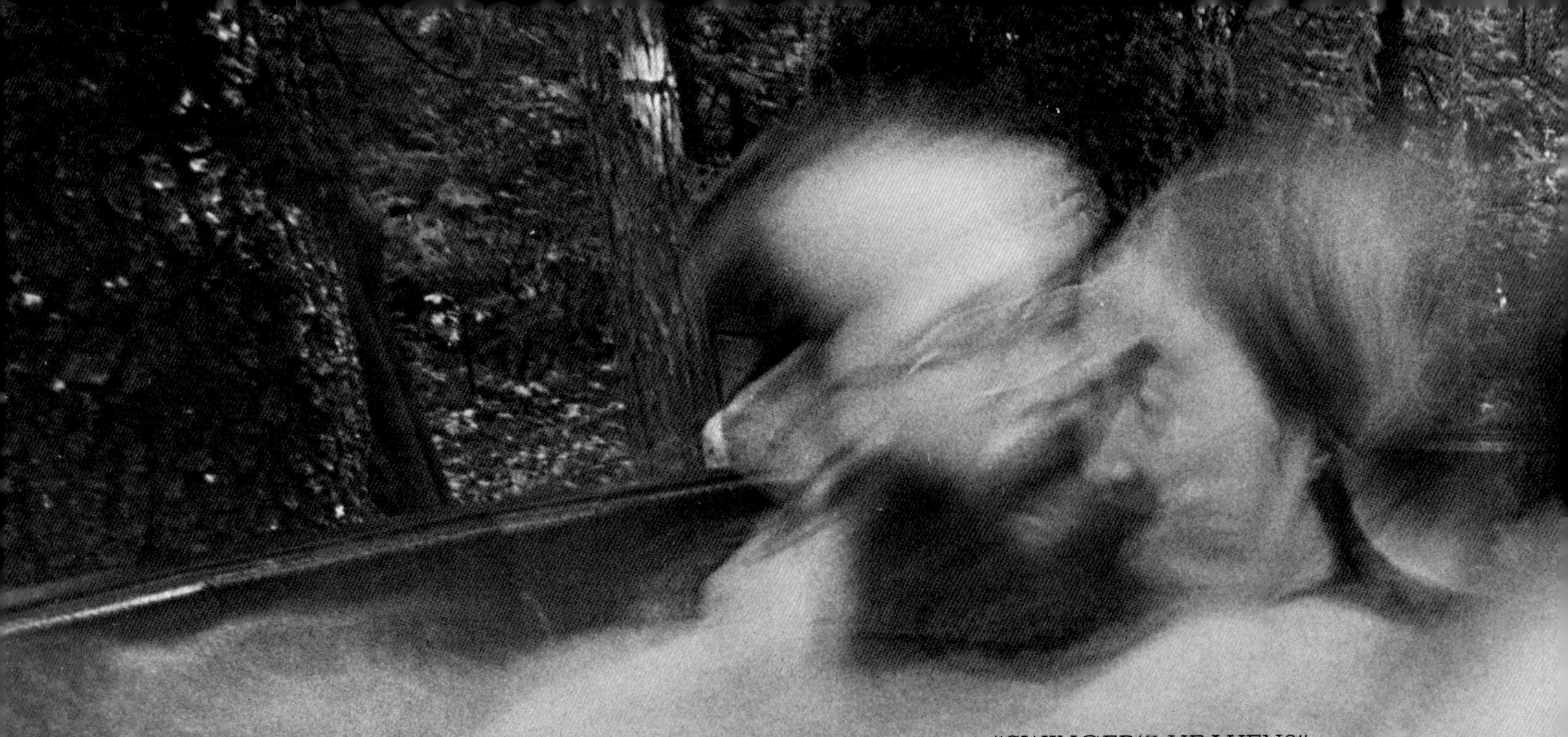

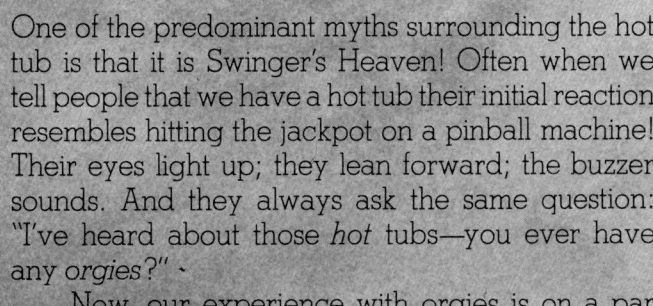

"SWINGER'S HEAVEN?"

One of the predominant myths surrounding the hot tub is that it is Swinger's Heaven! Often when we tell people that we have a hot tub their initial reaction resembles hitting the jackpot on a pinball machine! Their eyes light up; they lean forward; the buzzer sounds. And they always ask the same question: "I've heard about those *hot* tubs—you ever have any o*rgies*?"

Now, our experience with orgies is on a par with President Carter's sin of lust. We, too, have heard of hot tub parties where sexual activity abounds, but we've heard about it in bushes, on beaches and in bedrooms, too. Certainly nudity and sensuality are a natural part of hot tubbing, but simply owning a hot tub does not necessarily give you a passkey to lasciviousness. As in any location, to have an orgy, you need willing participants. And to have an orgy you don't have to have a hot tub.

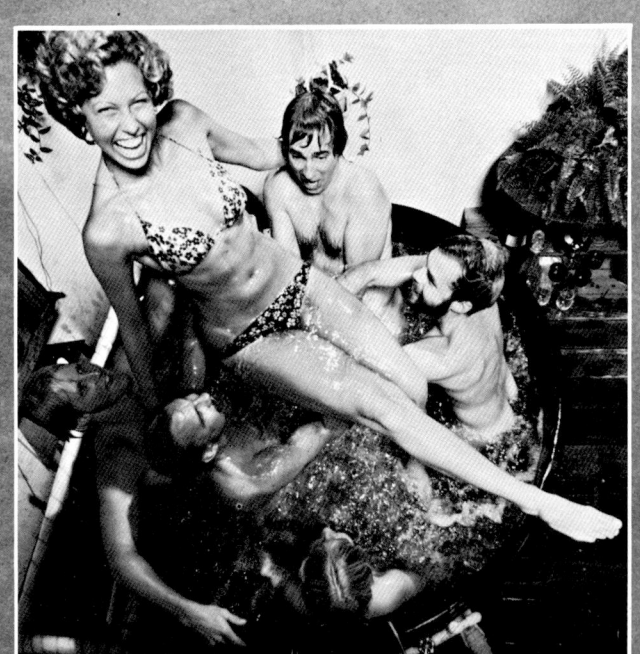

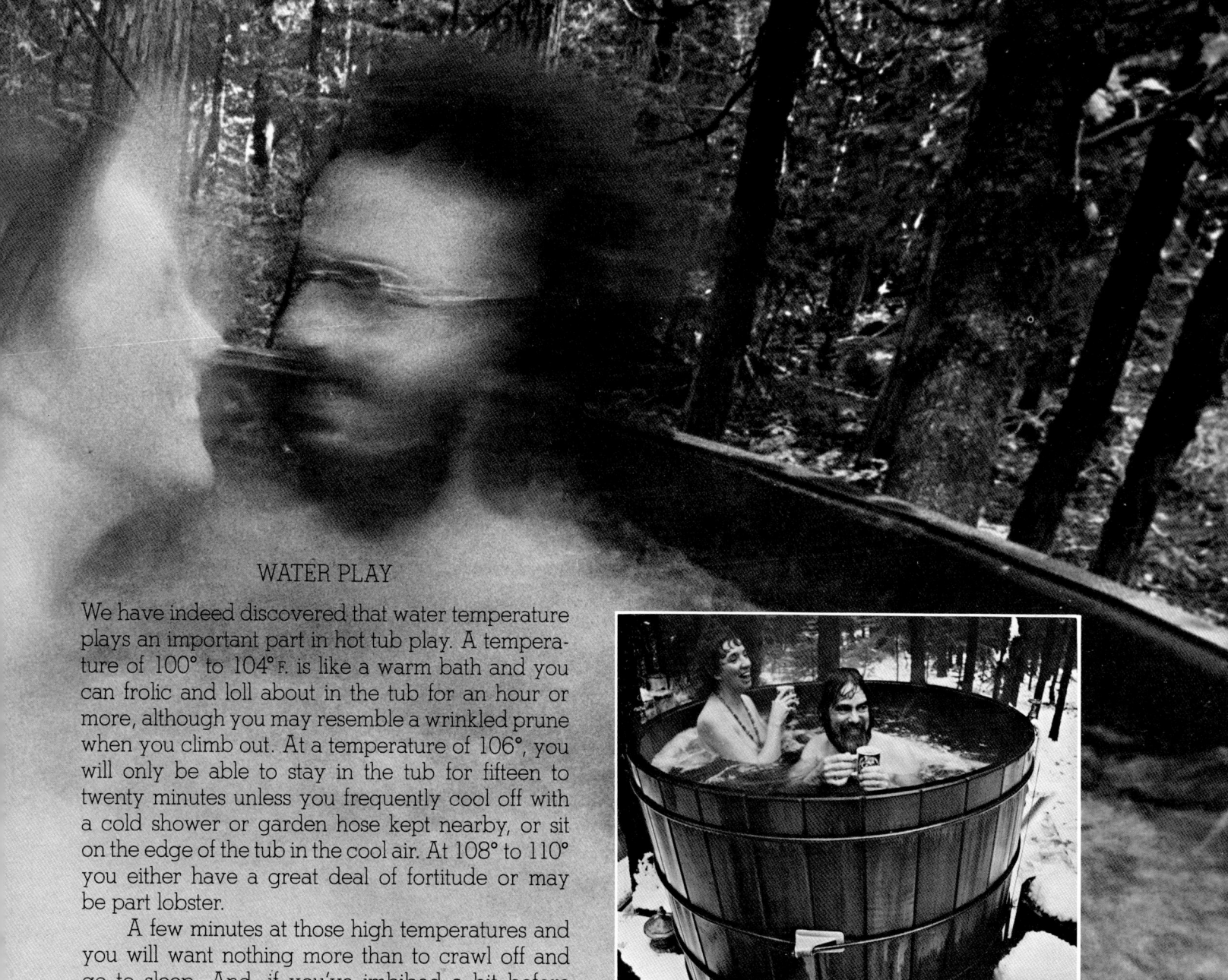

WATER PLAY

We have indeed discovered that water temperature plays an important part in hot tub play. A temperature of 100° to 104° F. is like a warm bath and you can frolic and loll about in the tub for an hour or more, although you may resemble a wrinkled prune when you climb out. At a temperature of 106°, you will only be able to stay in the tub for fifteen to twenty minutes unless you frequently cool off with a cold shower or garden hose kept nearby, or sit on the edge of the tub in the cool air. At 108° to 110° you either have a great deal of fortitude or may be part lobster.

    A few minutes at those high temperatures and you will want nothing more than to crawl off and go to sleep. And, if you've imbibed a bit before your bath, you'll probably need help crawling! So gauge your intentions as well as your water temperature, or you will find your romantic evening has turned into snores!

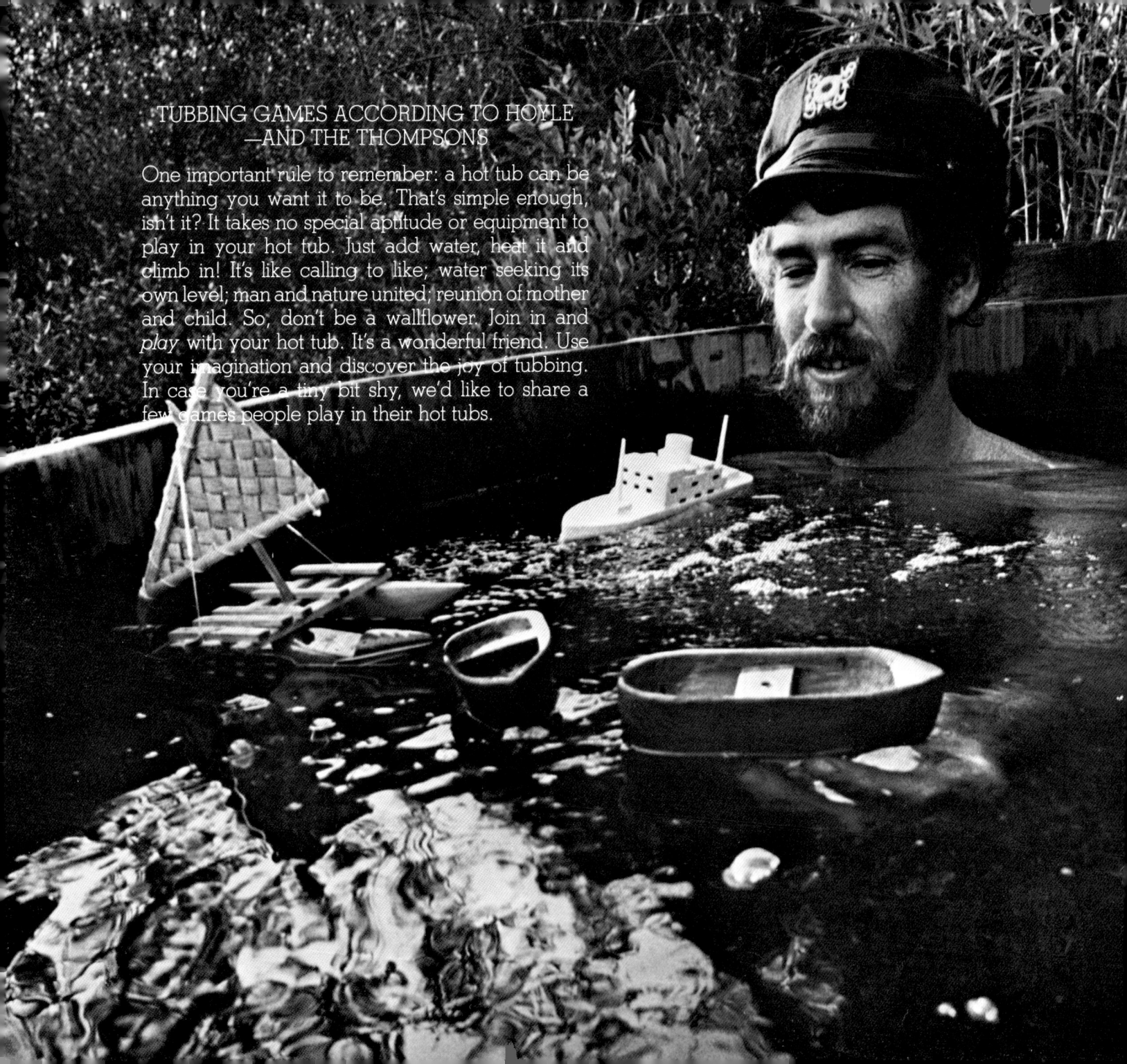

TUBBING GAMES ACCORDING TO HOYLE —AND THE THOMPSONS

One important rule to remember: a hot tub can be anything you want it to be. That's simple enough, isn't it? It takes no special aptitude or equipment to play in your hot tub. Just add water, heat it and climb in! It's like calling to like; water seeking its own level; man and nature united; reunion of mother and child. So, don't be a wallflower. Join in and *play* with your hot tub. It's a wonderful friend. Use your imagination and discover the joy of tubbing. In case you're a tiny bit shy, we'd like to share a few games people play in their hot tubs.

Executive Think-Tank

If you are a harried executive who arrives home to gulp down two martinis before you can bear to speak to your family, this game is for you. If you are the tired homemaker who fixed those two martinis for your harried husband before you could bear to speak to him, this game is for you, too. In fact, this pastime is for anyone who needs time to relax and unwind. Instead of tossing down those martinis or pulling out your hair, tell the *kids* to watch the Six O'clock News, and *you* go out and play!

Go climb into your hot tub together. First turn the air jets on for a few minutes and aim them at your aching neck and back muscles. Let yourself unwind. Then, when you realize you've stopped gritting your teeth, it's time to play "Executive Think-Tank."

Now, just let yourself go limp and float on the top of the water by leaning your head back on one edge of the tub, and hook your toes on the other side (if your tub is too large maneuver yourself until you can reach both sides). Next, close your eyes and let your mind wander. Follow the stream wherever it leads you. Think of pleasant thoughts; think of the most outrageous things you can. Don't block it—let yourself go. Your unconscious mind is full of wonderful things and rich memories. Let them come to you. You'll be surprised how your worries and tensions disappear and make room for your

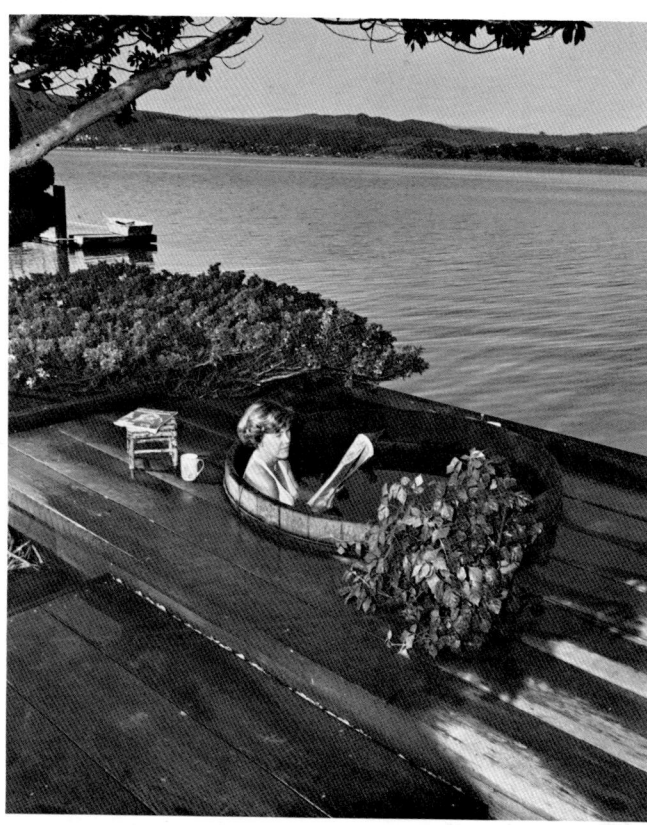

"mindless" wanderings. And, who knows, you might discover how to build the better mousetrap. Your conscious mind has simply been too cluttered and tense to tell you these things before.

Even if you don't revolutionize the world with your think-tank thoughts, you will discover a new formula: H_2O = RELAXATION + BLISS. Now, go back into the house and say hello to your kids and enjoy your evening!

"Any executive who plays with beer cans and toy boats in a hot tub has got to have a lot of class," says our friend on the left.

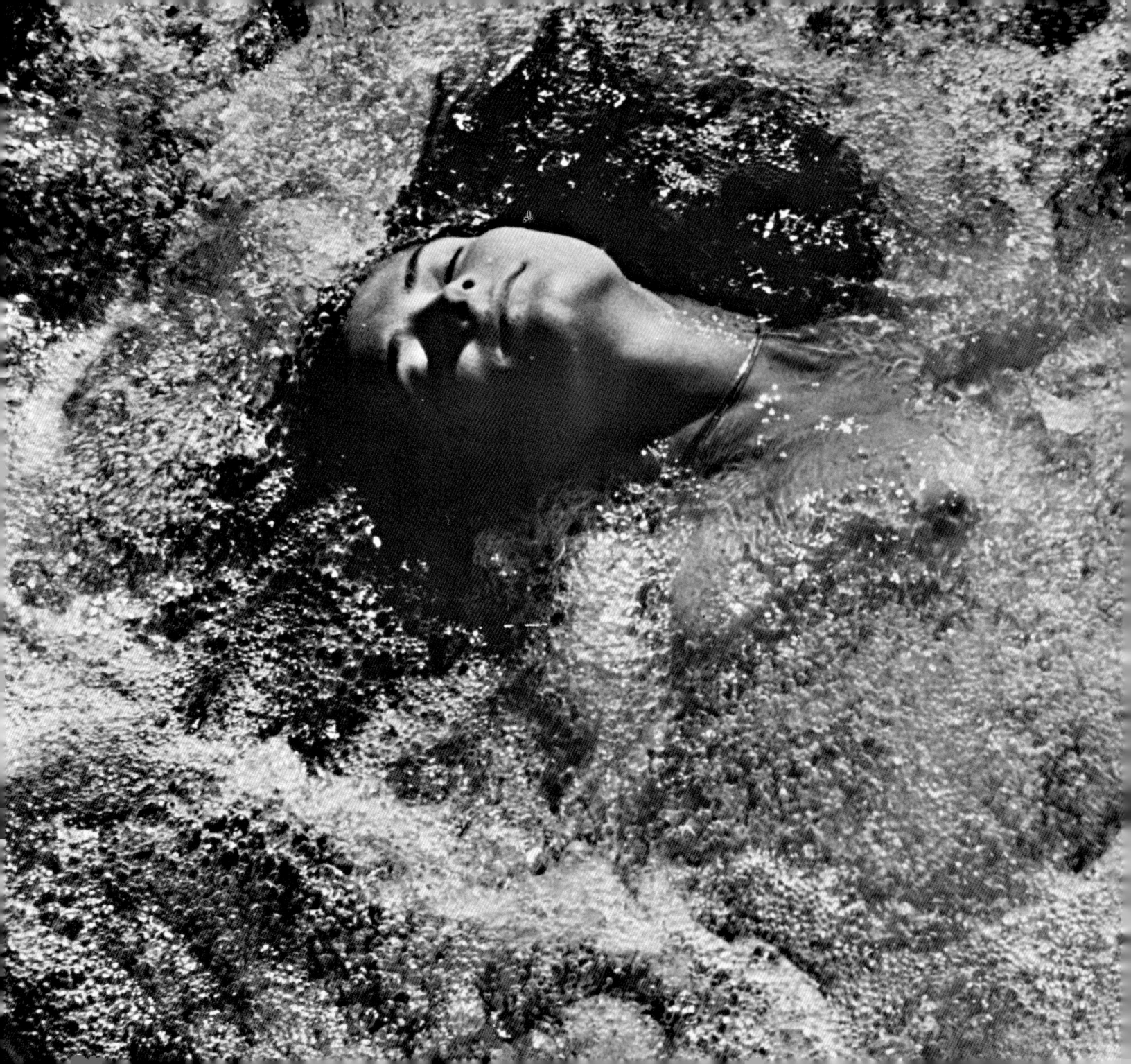

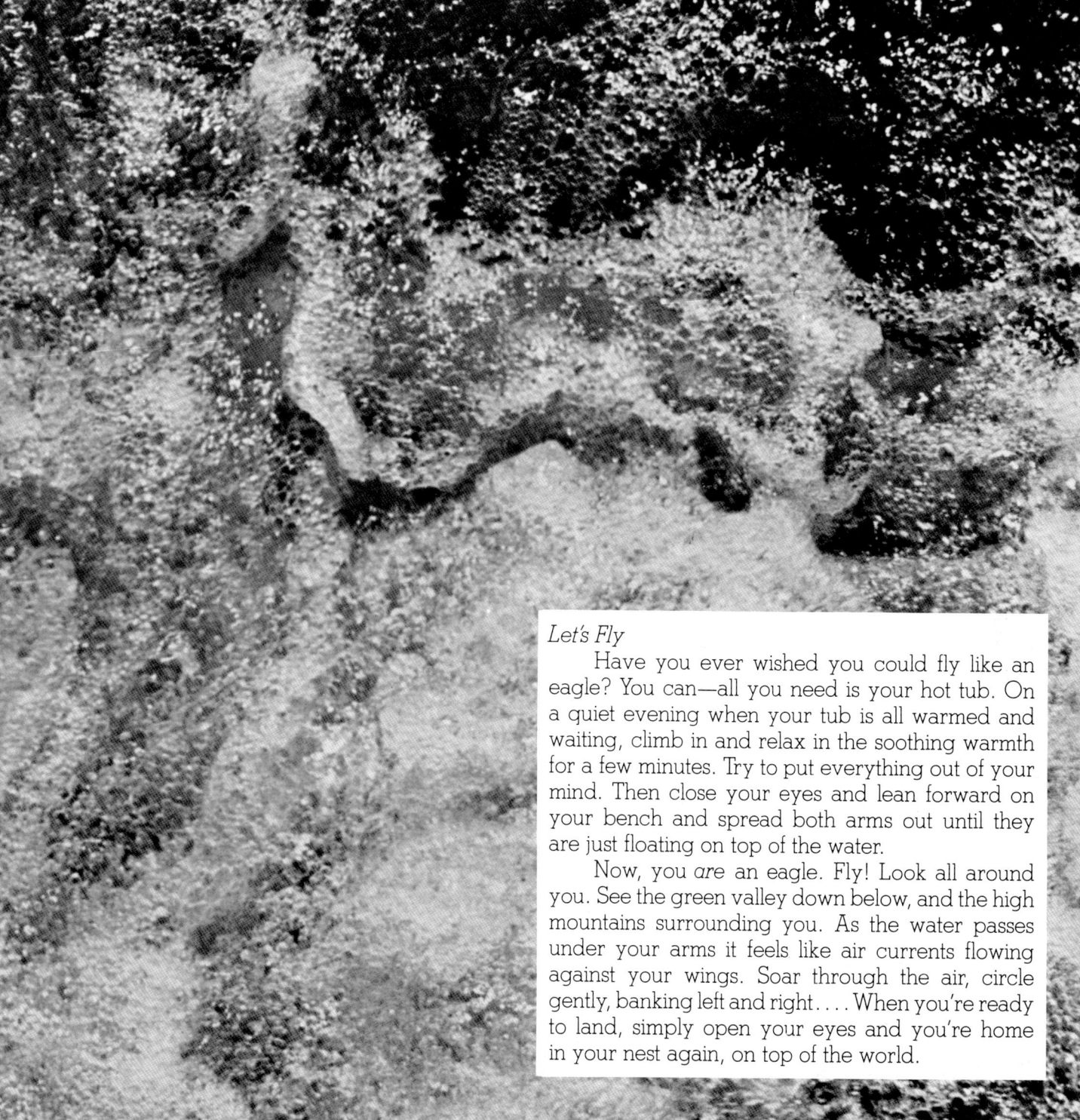

Let's Fly

Have you ever wished you could fly like an eagle? You can—all you need is your hot tub. On a quiet evening when your tub is all warmed and waiting, climb in and relax in the soothing warmth for a few minutes. Try to put everything out of your mind. Then close your eyes and lean forward on your bench and spread both arms out until they are just floating on top of the water.

Now, you *are* an eagle. Fly! Look all around you. See the green valley down below, and the high mountains surrounding you. As the water passes under your arms it feels like air currents flowing against your wings. Soar through the air, circle gently, banking left and right.... When you're ready to land, simply open your eyes and you're home in your nest again, on top of the world.

CANNIBAL SOUP

Your Own Fantasy Talk Show

One game we particularly like to play with new guests is to ask them to choose three or four people they'd like to share the hot tub with, and why. This is a great icebreaker, and once you've eliminated the more obvious choices like Robert Redford or Raquel Welch, you're likely to discover some really imaginative and revealing choices among your fellow hot tubbers.

One friend, a secret opera buff, surprised us with a first choice of Beverly Sills to join her in the bubbles (pun intended). We also discovered new insights into our politically conservative neighbor when he mulled over his choices and then announced: "Woody Allen, Jane Fonda and Dennis Banks."

We were delighted by another friend who grouped Mel Brooks, Bob Dylan, Johnny Carson and Orson Welles. Then he went on to imitate all of them in every hysterical detail, complete with Bob Dylan and Mel Brooks in musical serenade. While Dylan played *Lay, Lady, Lay,* on his harmonica, Mel Brooks munched Raisinets and sang *The Times, They Are A-Changin'* in a loud voice, almost drowning out Johnny Carson in the middle, trying to moderate the disaster by interjecting some of his famous one-liners. In the background, Orson Welles sat chest-high in the water, calmly holding a candle aloft and reading aloud from one of his filmscripts. This scene kept us laughing for hours.

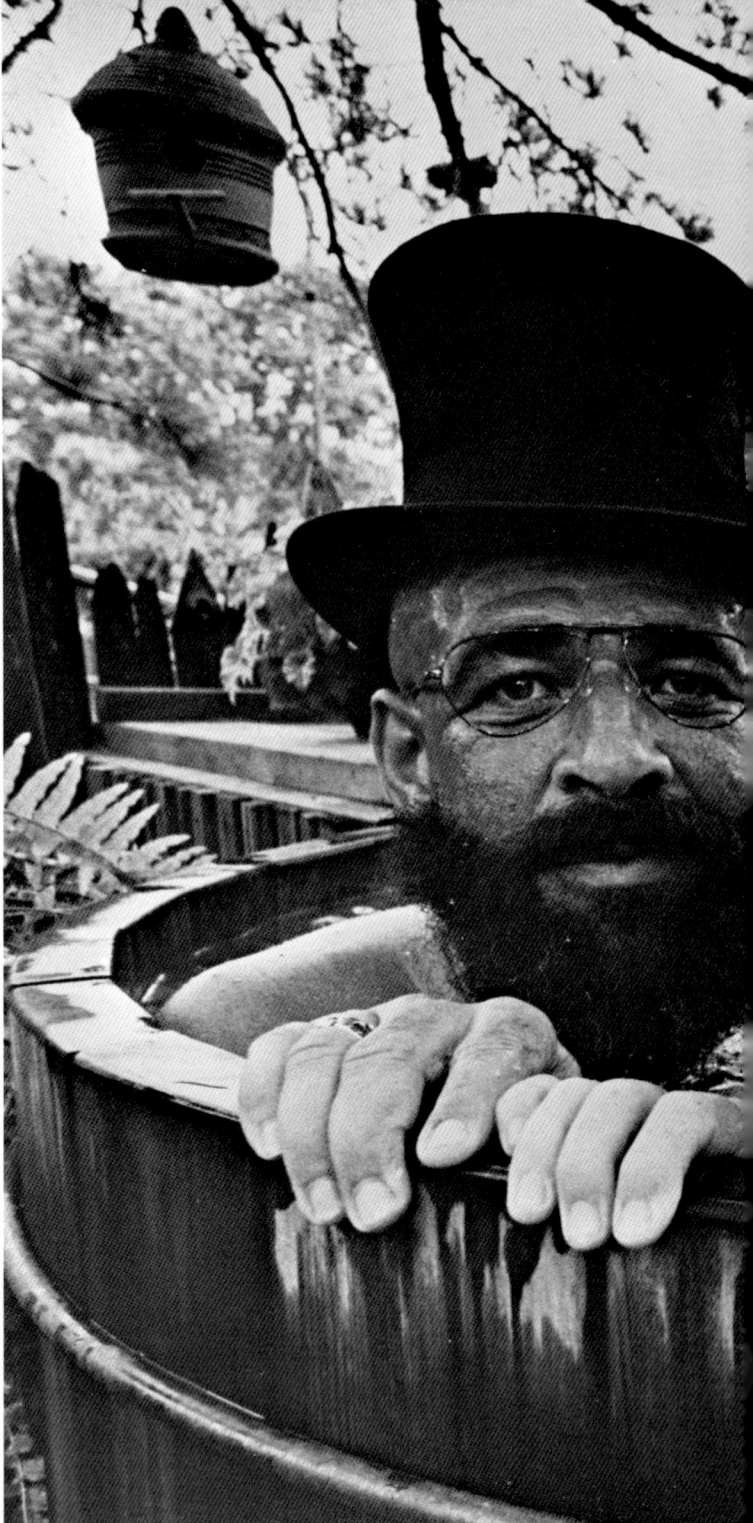

All dressed up for a night in the round.

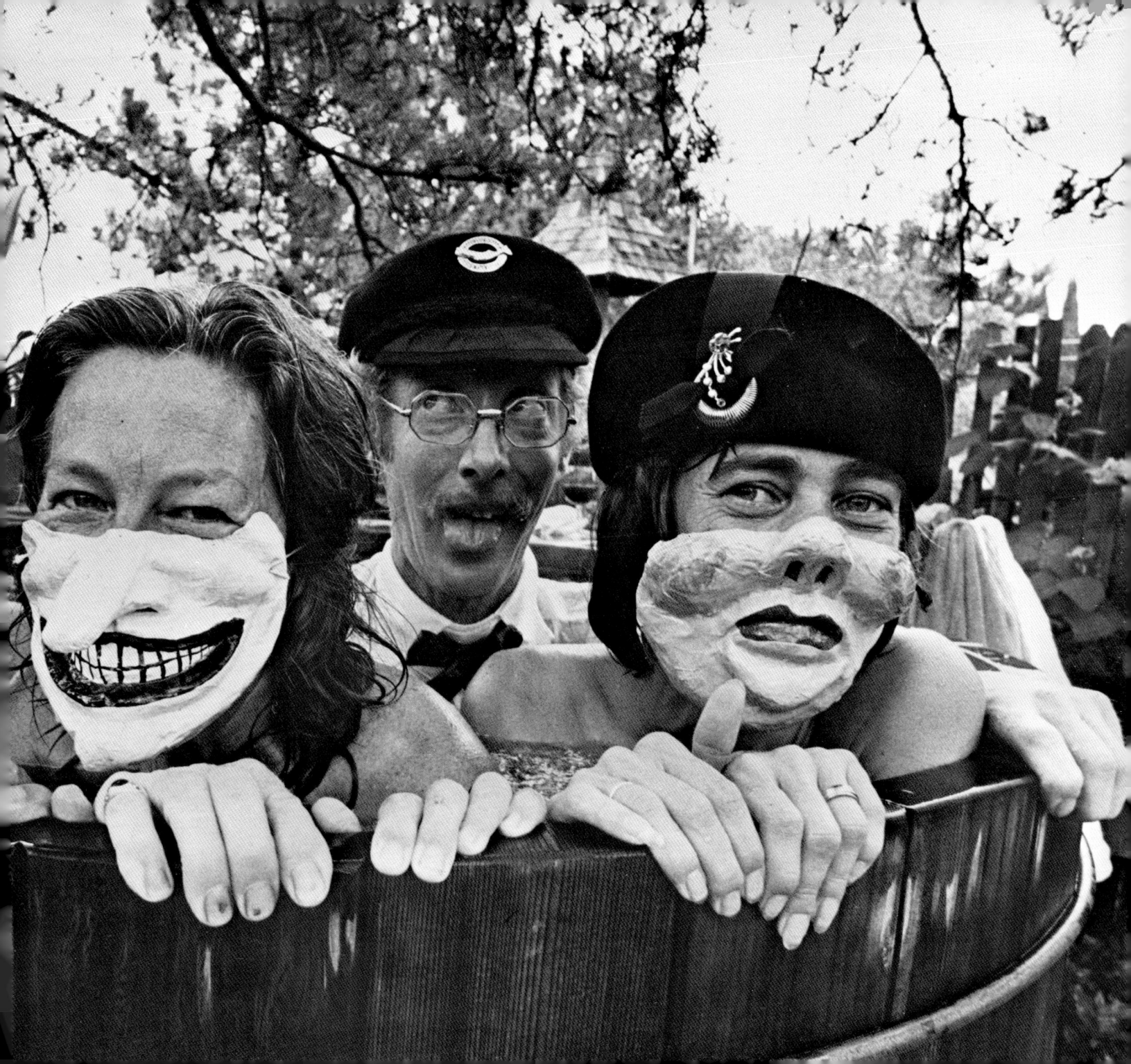

Star Gazing

A hot tub can be your own miniature observatory. All you need is a pair of eyes and a warm tub. Did you know the sky puts on its own show every night of the year? How many times have you made an effort to catch this Big Event? If you're like most people, probably not very often—perhaps once a year when you go camping, or as you walk to your house from your car. After all, when the astronomy guides tell you to bundle up and go outside and sit in a chair and stare at the sky all night, it doesn't sound very cozy.

Instead, imagine yourself soaking in hot, bubbling water up to your chin, with a sliver of a moon and millions of stars overhead. . . . What a way to study astronomy!

As you view those twinkling stars from your vantage point in the steamy tub, you will find yourself wondering why a certain grouping of stars has moved from where they seemed to be the night before. Soon you begin to realize that the stars are in a different spot in the sky at different hours of the evening. Next, you begin to wonder why you've never bothered to learn the names of all those configurations. They've been up there all your life and you've never learned more than the Big Dipper, the Little Dipper, and the North Star.

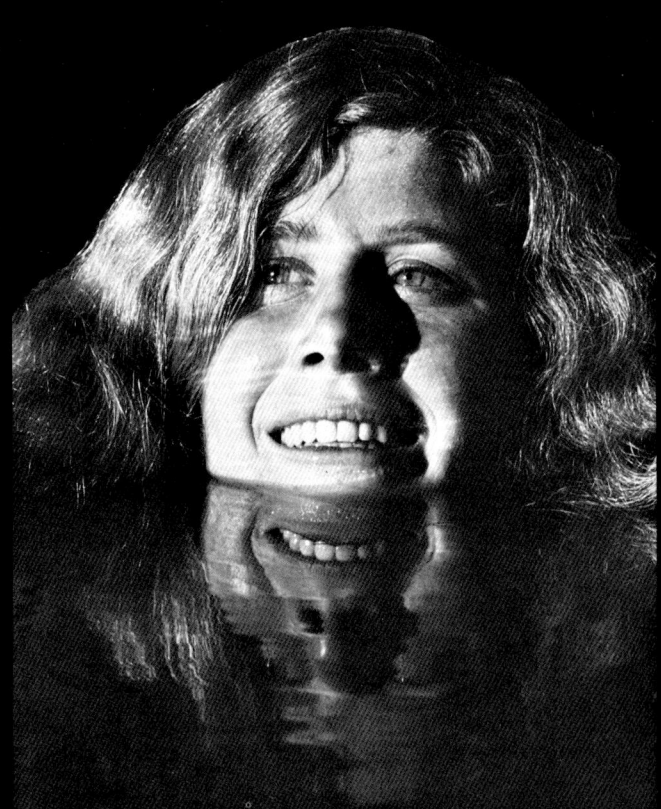

Once you have whetted your appetite and become familiar with the brightest stars and most important constellations, you may want to increase your knowledge of the stars by purchasing a beginner's guide to astronomy. Begin by learning the names and locations of the major constellations. As soon as it gets dark, you can spot the most visible stars and planets without the aid of a telescope or field glasses. All you need is your eyes. As the earth rotates and new stars become visible in the eastern sky, you can add to your knowledge. Any beginner's guide to stars will provide you with seasonal star charts and directions for locating the heavenly bodies.

Your initial feeling of wonder and thrill of recognition will increase as you study the stars through night after night observation, all the while sitting comfortably in your warm armchair—the hot tub.

Hot Tub Myths and Fantasies

STAR GAZING

Lay your head back
And look at those stars
See them twinkle
Hello in the night.
Were they always there
And we never noticed?
Was the smog so thick?
We couldn't see?
Or are we now looking
For the beauty in things,
Instead of just looking
To see?
    John Thompson

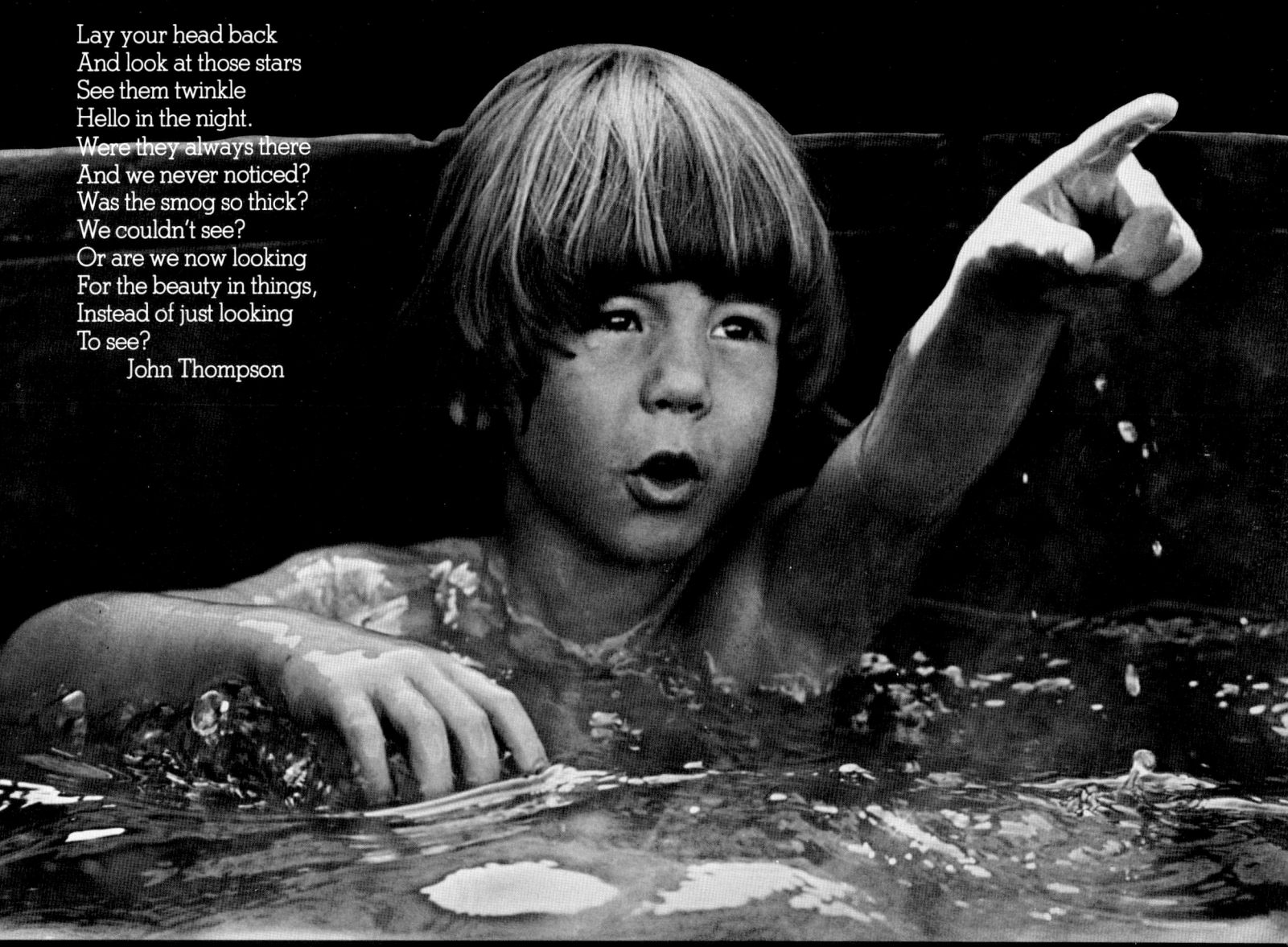

CANNIBAL SOUP

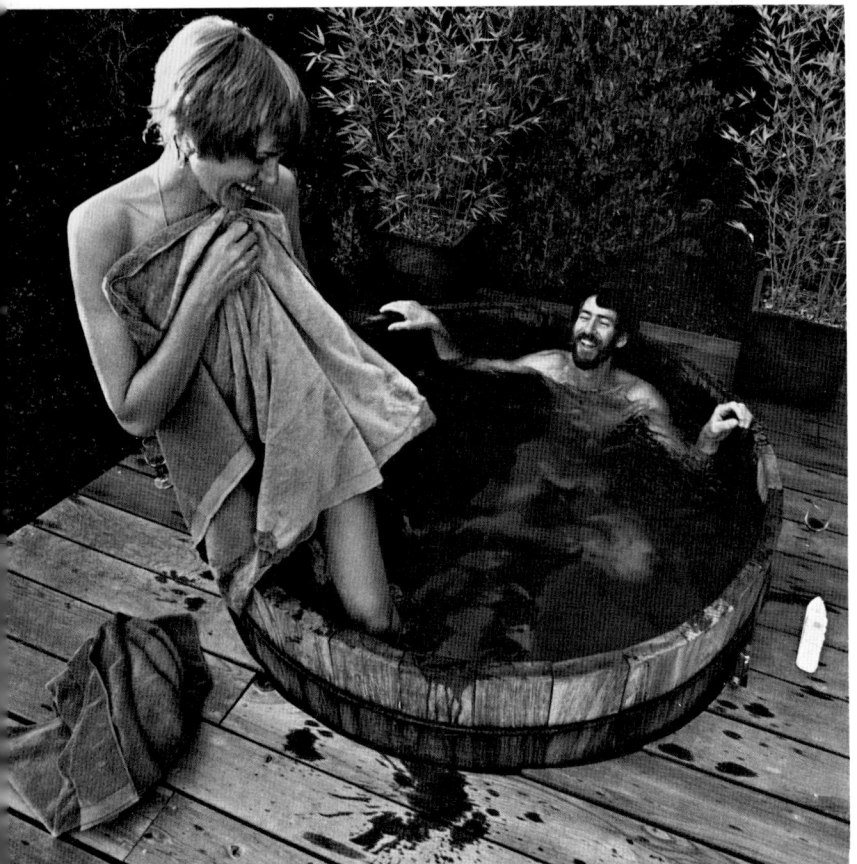

DOING IT RIGHT

Now that we have explored some hot-tub myths and fantasies, a few words about the amenities of tubbing. First, you'll find that there is nothing nicer than slipping into a soft terrycloth robe after a relaxing session in your hot tub. Now, a terrycloth robe doesn't sound very chic, but you'll find your Pierre Cardin silk lounging robe will feel like a sheet of ice against your warm skin. Then you'll tense up and destroy all the beneficial effects of the minutes spent lounging in the tub. Forsake fad, fashion and trend—stick to good old terrycloth.

Next, supply your guests with fresh, dry towels when they step out of the hot tub. There's nothing worse than trying to dry off with a clammy, already-been-used towel. You don't have to go out and splurge on large beach towels for a dozen guests—a regular bath towel will get your guests just as dry and happy.

Finally, try adding mineral bath salts for an extra treat for you and your guests. You can buy a jar of salts such as *Batherapy* from health food stores or drugstores. These are concentrated bath salts containing minerals similar to those in famous hot springs and spas all over the world. In addition to soothing your aching muscles, they add a bit of color and scent to your hot tub. We especially like salts that smell like the pines that surround our tub. Don't be afraid to be a bit adventurous—this isn't your porcelain bathtub we're talking about. A hot tub is a whole new way of life!

Simple terrycloth is transformed into a luxurious fabric designed to keep the body's warmth in after a relaxing soak in 105° water.

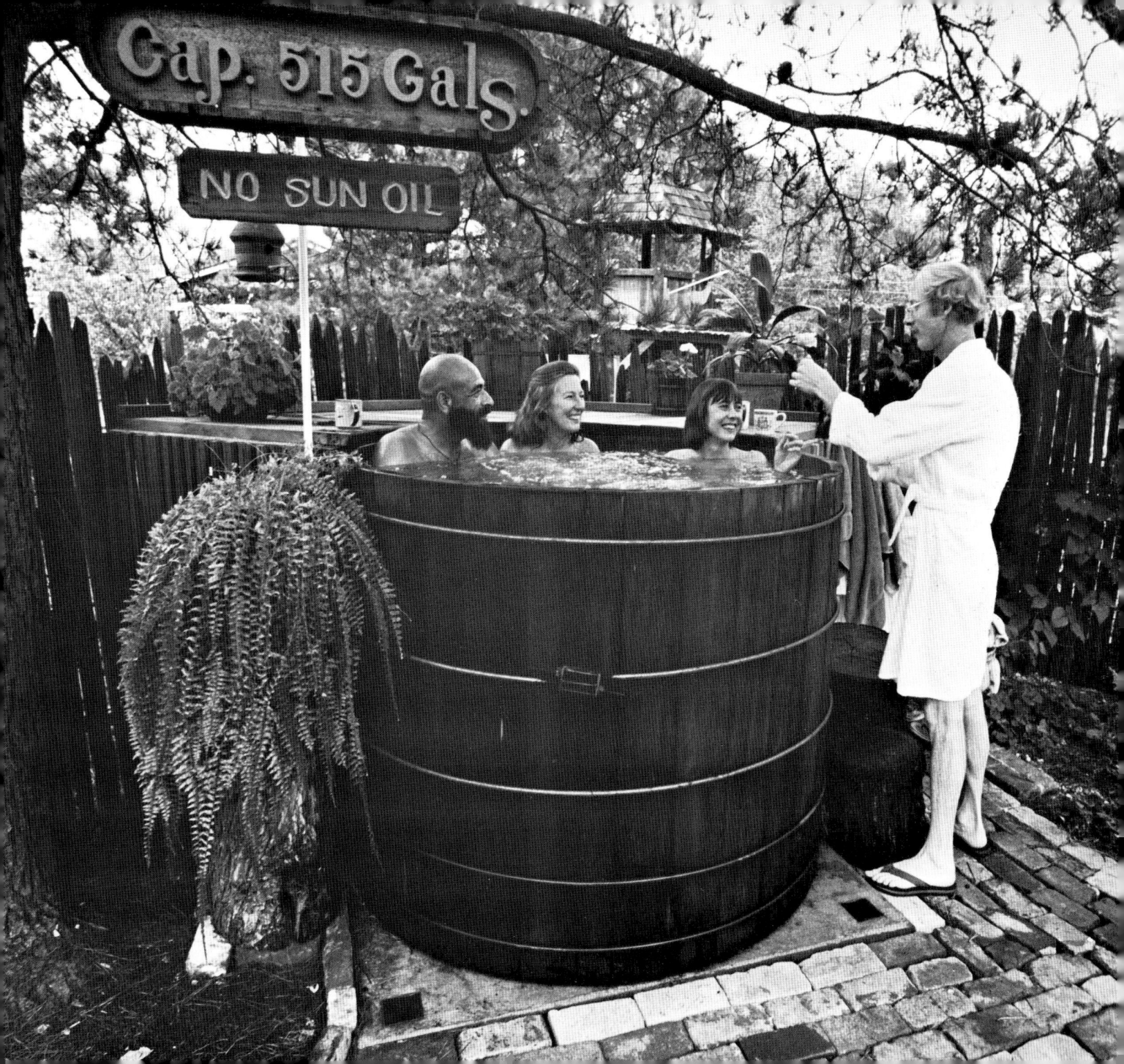

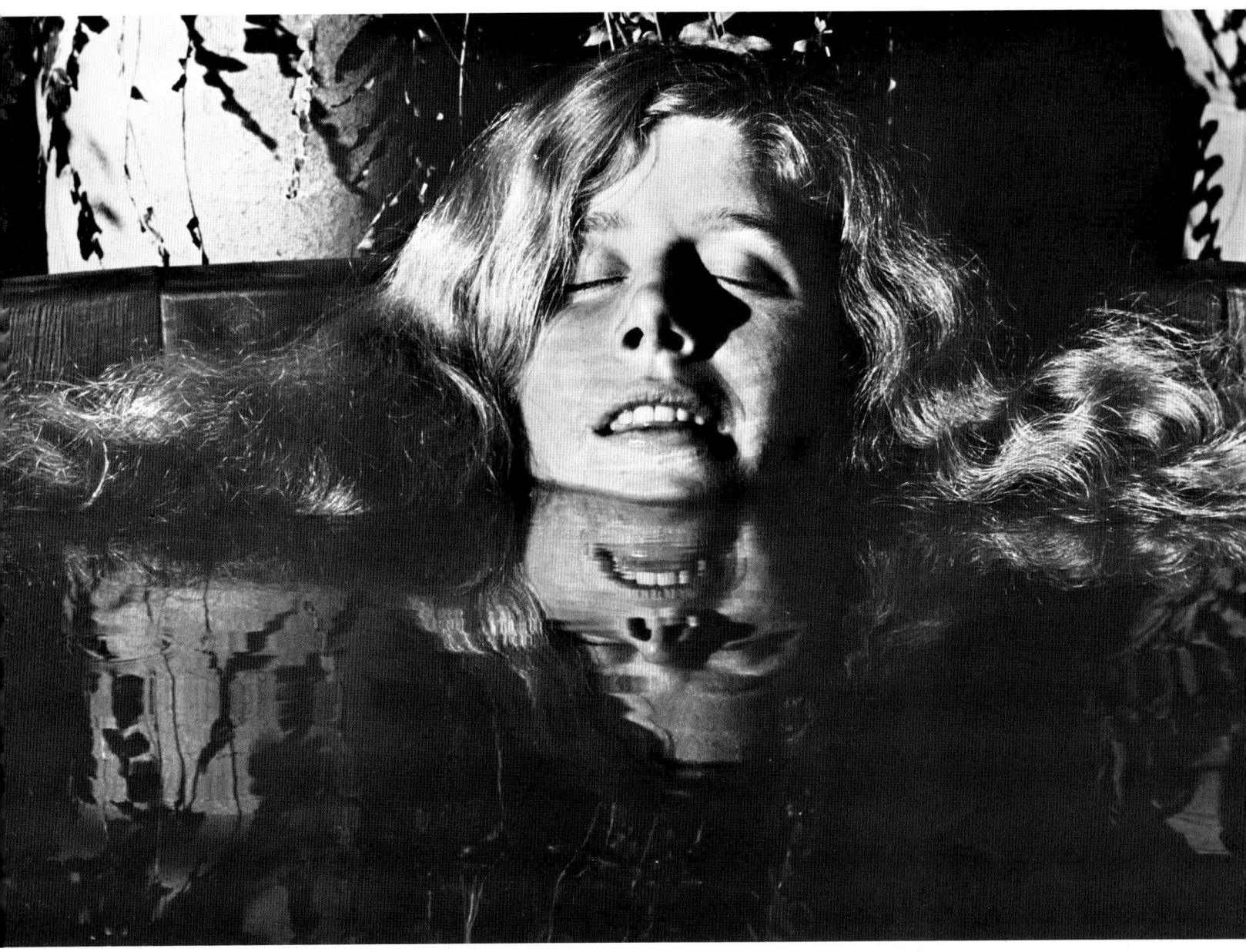

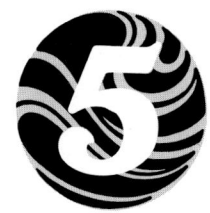

THROW THOSE SLEEPING PILLS AWAY!

Tick-tock, tick-tock; midnight, one o'clock, two o'clock, three, and you still can't sleep. You've tried counting sheep. You've commanded your muscles to relax, one by one. Instead, you lie awake wrestling with your budget, trying to balance a 6 percent cost-of-living raise against a 15 percent raise in the cost of living. Finally, tense and irritable, you reach for a sleeping pill, knowing you're going to pay for it in the morning when the alarm forces you groggily out of bed to face the looming day.

Sound familiar? It should; doctors prescribe more tranquilizers today than any other drug. And the makers of the other "safe and restful" sleeping aids are not exactly facing bankruptcy. We are one nation democratically united under pressure; pressure of the people, by the people, and for the people.

There's no escape, so we cope with it as best we can. The phone book is full of psychiatrists and self-certified therapists. The liquor industry has never been in better spirits. Young people and old are embracing new religions and/or new drugs. Self-help books are selling like hot cakes. In the past decades we have learned of EST, transcendental meditation, transactional analysis, bio-feedback and inner-awareness, the primal scream. All promise a better way to cope with everyday life.

We are a nation spending millions of dollars on a better way of life. We buy recreational vehicles to escape the crush of the city only to crawl bumper-to-bumper for hours on the freeway, and then check into a roadside camp full of other haggard RV campers. We make long-term reservations to swim or boat on a public lake or to visit a national park. Skiing is eternal lines of cars on the highways, lines for the lifts, lines for the *après* ski drinks. Tennis courts and golf courses are first-come, first-served. Airports are teeming lines of jostling travelers, with even airplanes in lines in the sky, forced to wait in holding patterns before landing. It's no wonder we all stagger back to work to rest up from our vacation.

Wouldn't it be wonderful to enjoy your leisure time in a leisurely manner, rid yourself of tension, and get a good night's sleep every night? You can—all you need is a hot tub . . . a fountain of youth right in your own backyard. So throw away those sleeping pills, break the bad news to your liquor store, tell Werner Erhard what you *really* think of him, and prepare to be the most relaxed, devil-may-care person around. Ponce de Leon—you just didn't look long enough to find it.

JUST WHAT THE DOCTOR ORDERED!

As you learn more about hot tubs you will hear a lot about *hydrotherapy*. Don't let this technical term put you off. *Hydro* means water, and *pathy,* a system of treating disease or illness. So *hydrotherapy* and *hydropathy* simply mean you feel better through the use of water. Professional athletes have been soaking their aches and pains through the use of hydromassage and hydrotherapy for years.

Your hot tub comes equipped with two or more hydrotherapy air inlets which direct pulsating streams of hot bubbling water to those aching spots on your body. The millions of massaging bubbles bouncing off your neck and back will do much more for your tired body than sleeping pills.

Ancient civilizations have long known the therapeutic benefits of the hot bath. Today's *beautiful people* jet all over the world to visit hot springs and spas to find hot mineral water to relieve their mental and physical tension.

Japanese legends abound with tales of wounded or injured animals and birds found recuperating after bathing in a hot spring; animals instinctively

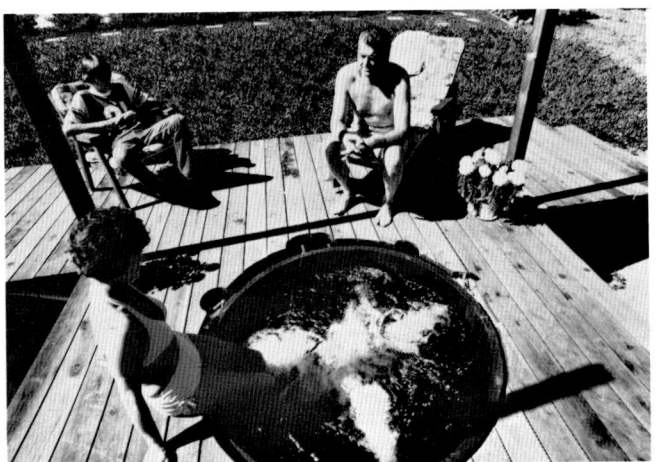

Baseball Great, Don Larsen, finds his hot tub the perfect relaxer.

sought out the curative powers of mineral waters even before man discovered their healthful benefits. The famous waters of Bath, in Southwestern England, offered cures for a wide range of diseases such as arthritis, lumbago, organic nervous disorders, circulatory disturbances, female disorders—and even obesity!

Here is a simple example of the curative powers of the hot tub. A friend of ours slipped and fell while indulging in some horseplay, and landed with his foot twisted beneath him. Immediately, his ankle swelled and he could barely hobble about. He climbed into our hot tub and spent the rest of the afternoon in and out of the hot water. The next morning his ankle was back to normal and he didn't have a shadow of a bruise!

Foremost on the list of healthful benefits offered by any hot tub or spa, are the ones we as a nation are most troubled with: general malaise; lack of

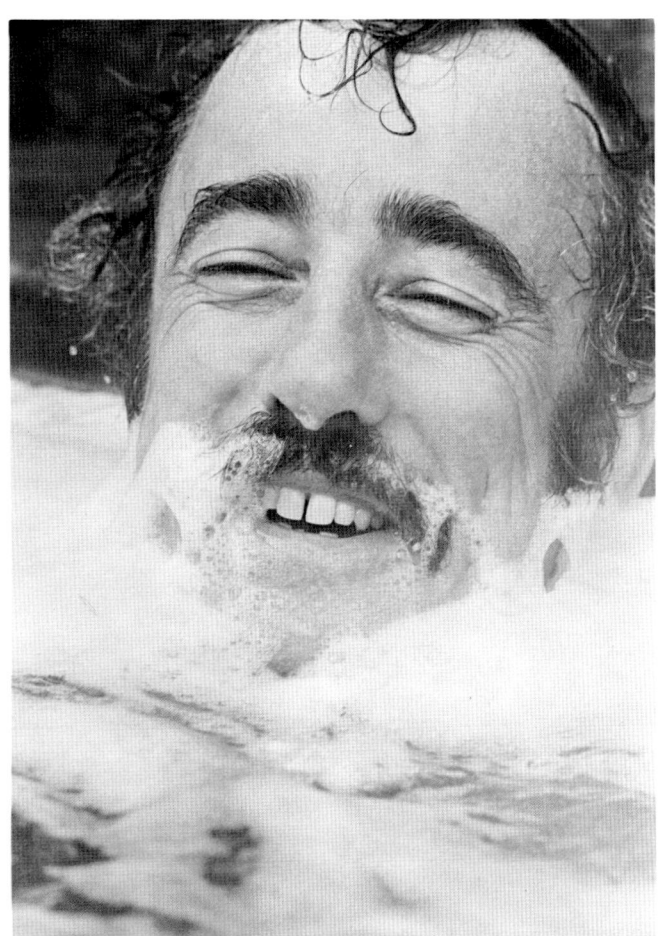 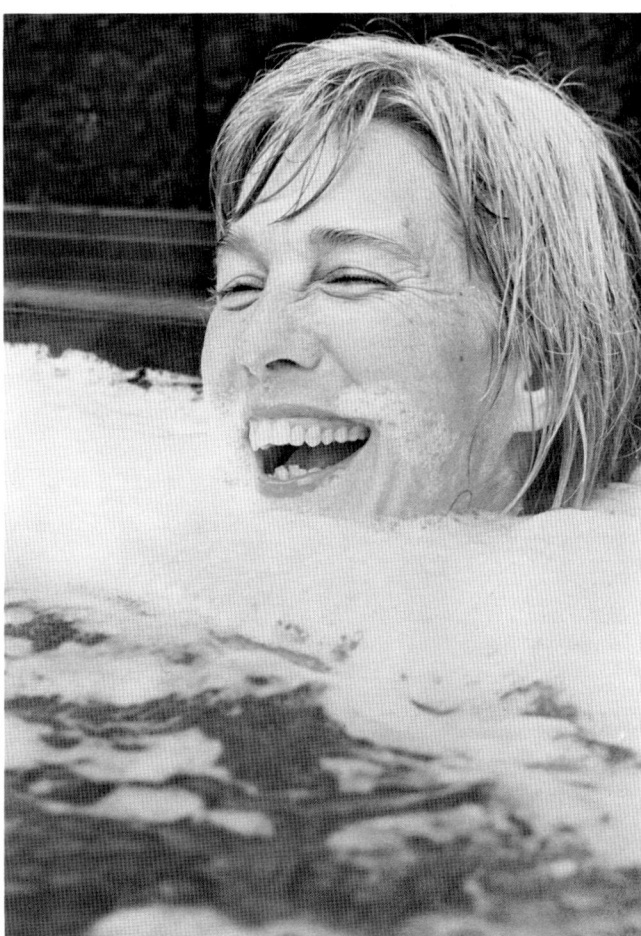

A little foam never hurt anybody! Excess foaming is sometimes caused by newly added chlorine in conjunction with vigorous hydrotherapy jets.

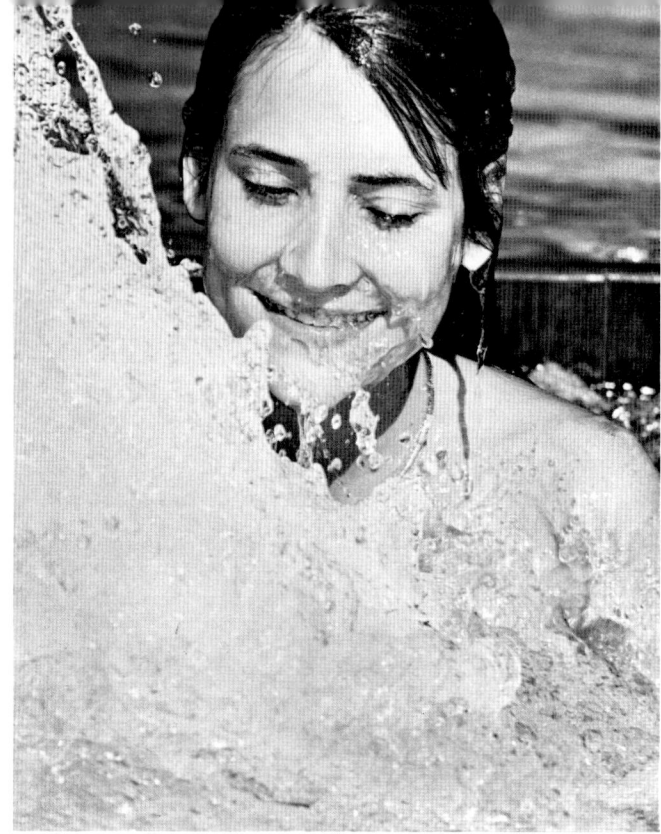
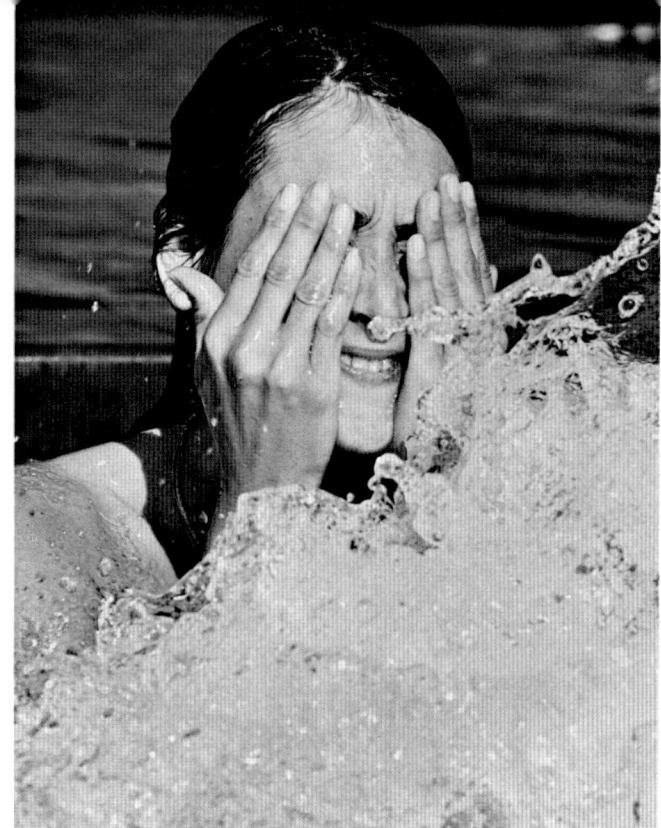

muscle tone; insomnia; tension. Because of its value in treating these everyday problems, the hot tub is said to be the single most effective method of promoting well-being and alleviating anxiety in this tension-ridden age!

CAUTION A hot tub is *not* a cure for all ailments. If you have a serious health problem, check with your doctor before jumping into a tub. If you have breathing difficulties such as emphysema, or if you have hardening of the arteries, or other coronary or circulatory diseases, a hot tub might not be a good thing. Hot, steamy water makes breathing more difficult for weakened lungs. It also creates a demand for blood to the heated areas of your body which might overwork the already over-burdened heart and/or arteries. Your hot-tub heater has a thermostat which can be set at a lower temperature to avoid aggravating these problems. As a lay expert on nutrition and health cautions:

The main danger with the hot tub is the hotness of the water for the extreme periods of time. You have to match temperature and duration of the bath to your own personal condition. If you get out of the tub and feel drained, you've been in too long—or it's too hot. Instead of being invigorating, it's enervating. It takes energy from the body. Moderation is the guide to all of these aids.

Cary Nosler

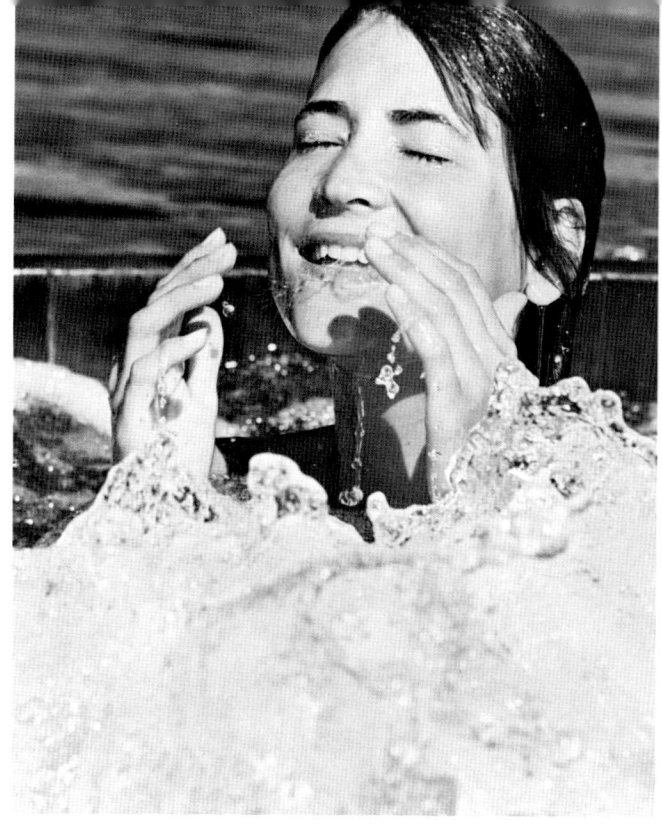 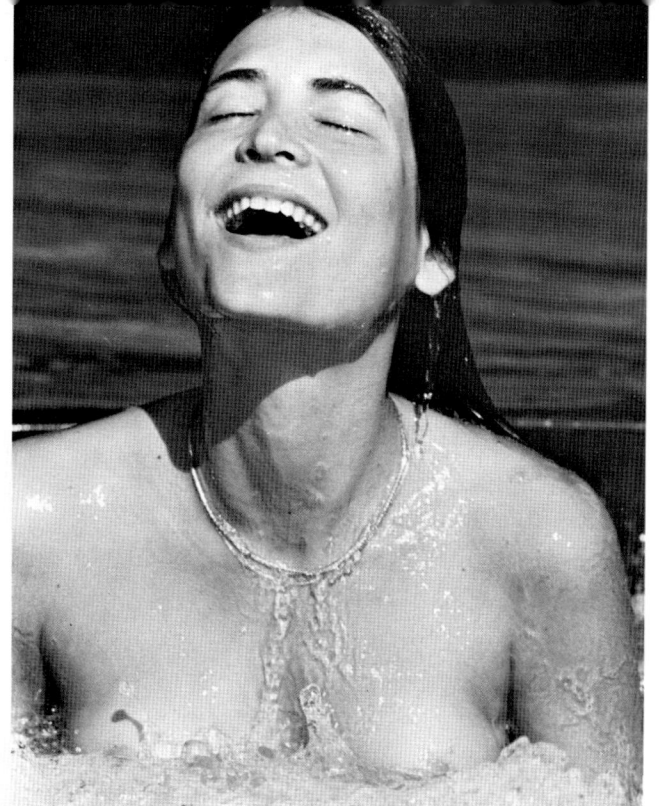

Warm water and invigorating bubbles—hydrotherapy doesn't have to be a drag!

So *do* consult with your physician first—after all, some people are even allergic to milk.

Our hot tub is the best investment we've made. But, along with the tub, we received an extra bonus—while filing our income taxes, we found we could deduct the cost of the tub from our medical expenses because it was prescribed by Valerie's doctor for treatment of phlebitis. The Internal Revenue Service says no two cases are the same, and they reserve the right to evaluate each case on its own merit, but if you, or someone in your family, has a *certifiable* health problem, and your doctor prescribes hydrotherapy treatment, you may be able to deduct the cost of your hot tub as a medical expense.

We talked to many doctors when we first became interested in a hot tub. Almost every one said, given a choice, he would rather prescribe a glass of wine and a session in a hot tub than a tranquilizer any day! It makes more sense to relax with a "natural" sedative than an addictive chemical substance, anyway. Life should be good, and a cause for personal celebration. So celebrate with something sensual and sensational—climb into your own therapeutic spa every night and enjoy a safe and restful sleep. Then get up in the morning ready to live.

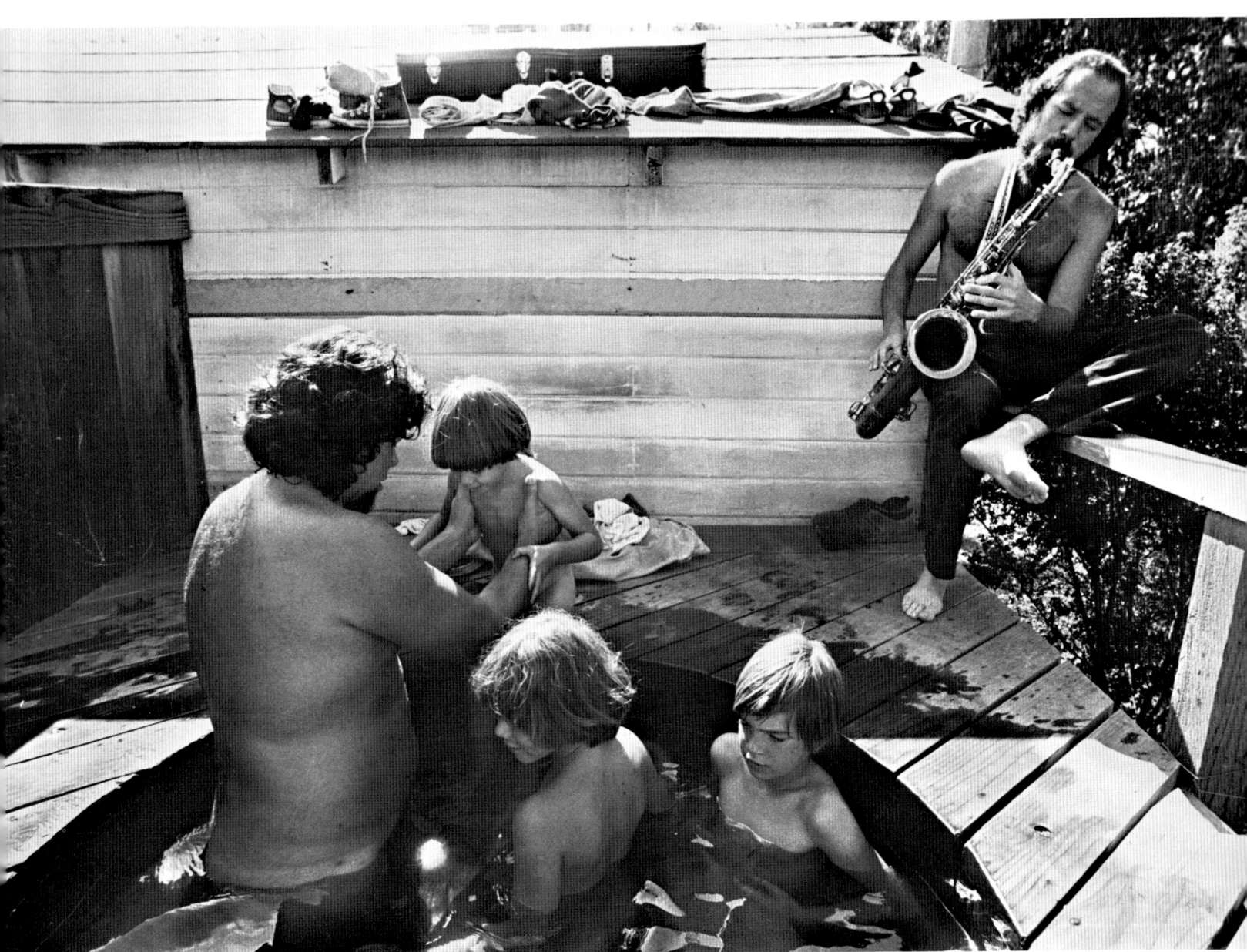

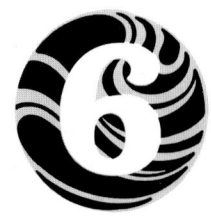

M-M-M-M-M-M-M-M-M-M-M

M is for a million things. Maybe you've always thought of the letter M as a mundane, middle-of-the-alphabet letter. We want to make M a Monumental Milestone—or at least a capital letter—in honor of the myriad moods M lends itself to.

MOZART, MICK JAGGER & MANTOVANI

Whatever your taste in music, you'll find that your hot tub is a natural concert hall. Some feel Handel's *Water Music* couldn't be more appropriate; we like Strauss waltzes or harpsichord music best. Somehow the soft melodic classics enhance the tranquility and reverie. But if Steve Miller or Mick Jagger make you feel alive and happy, feel free to indulge. Do give the classics a try, though, because if plants grow better, and cows give more milk while listening to Bach or Beethoven—who knows what might happen to you!

We're blessed with friends who can play various musical instruments, which often results in a jam session or a good ol' sing-along. But we don't advise a six-piece ensemble to join you in your tub, since a bass fiddle displaces too much water. The best way to enjoy a full band is to install stereo speakers near the tub and pipe those good sounds right outside to you. Then crank up the volume so it's agreeable to you *and* your neighbors and let the good times roll.

If no musical instruments are available, use your God-given ones—your own voices. An a cappella choir singing rounds of "Row, Row, Row Your Boat" is one of the greatest icebreakers we know. Friends made our Christmas special this year when they joined hands in the tub while their voices singing "Silent Night" drifted up through the trees and the falling snow.

CANNIBAL SOUP

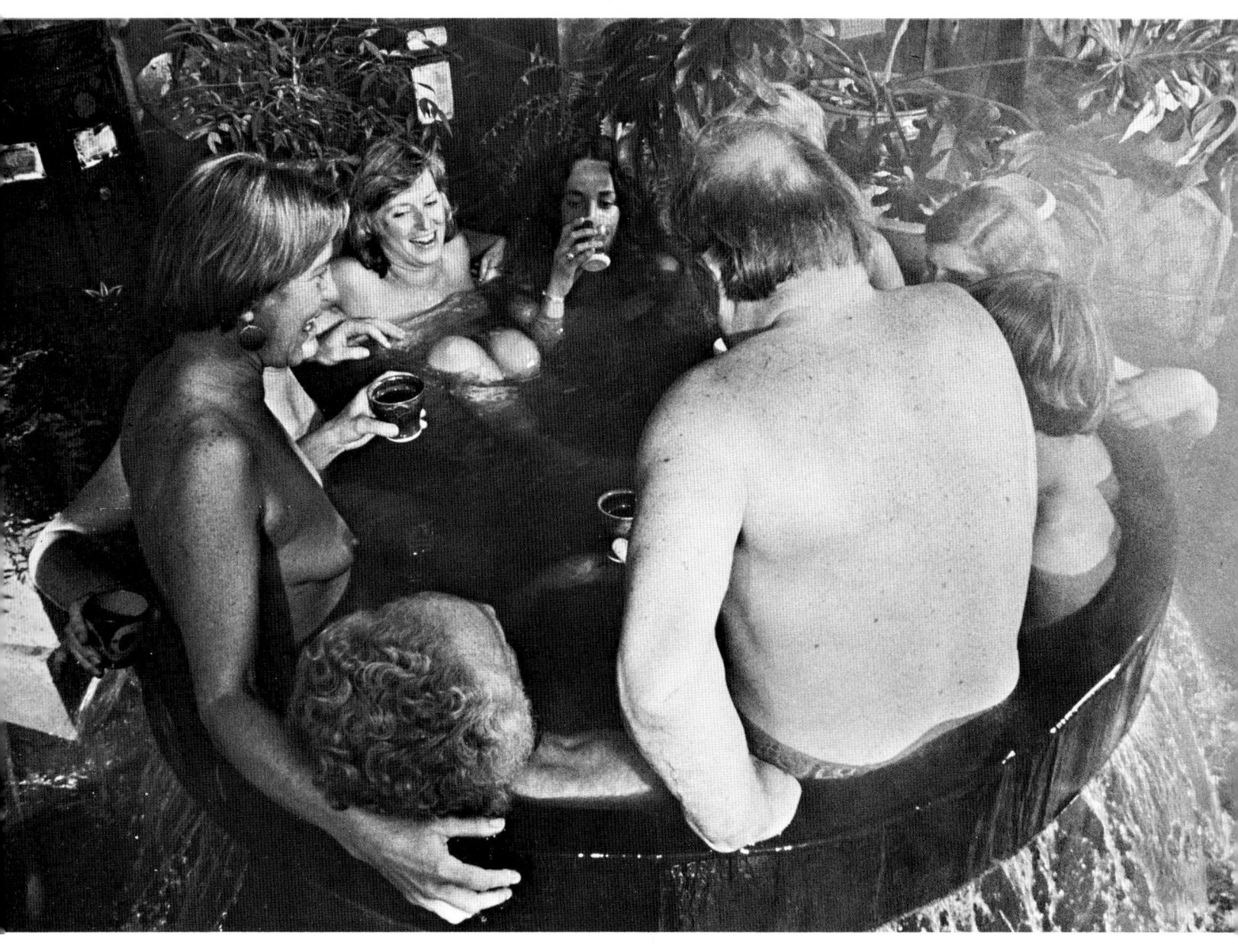

MARTINIS, MARGARITAS, & MONDAVI

Many of you are fond of your favorite mixed drink. We would like to caution you before you plunge into your hot tub after imbibing several highballs or martinis. The heat of the tub will send your circulation racing, and those few ounces of alcohol will suddenly seem like quarts! In other words, it will go to your head—quickly—leaving you unsteady, weak and *very* drunk. Moderation in mixed drinks is the key word here.

    Soon after our first experience crawling out of the tub wobbly kneed and stumbling to the nearest chair, we took the easy way out and switched to drinking wine before tubbing. A few glasses of jug wine or your favorite Mirrasou or Mondavi, will leave you relaxed, but still able to handle the hot water in the tub. And, you don't have to worry about throwing suddenly tipsy guests the life preserver.

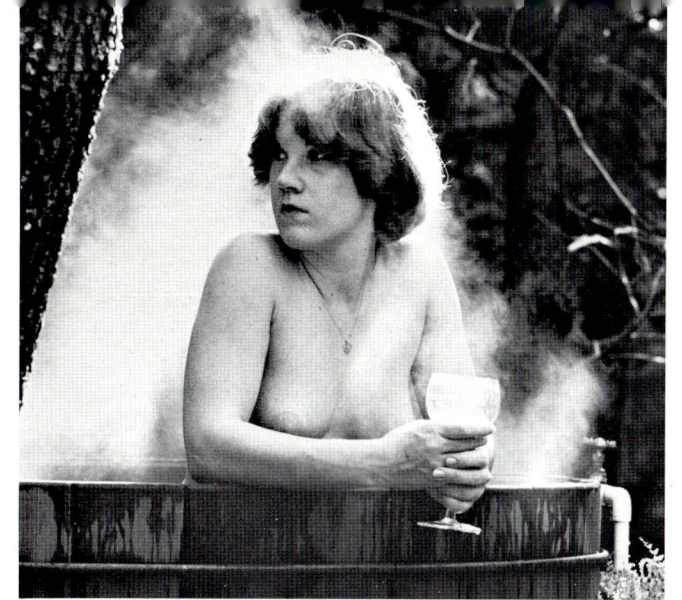

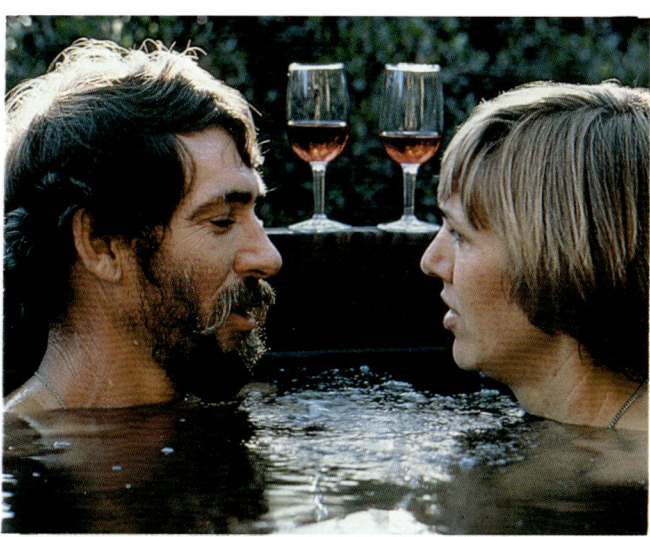

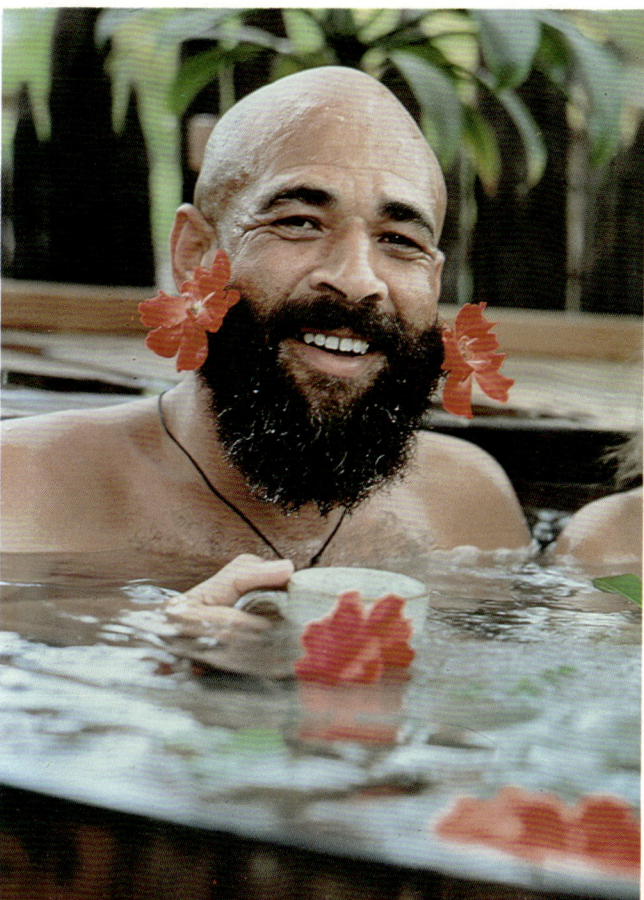

CANNIBAL SOUP

MOOD-ENHANCERS & MUNCHIES

Marijuana is a favorite mood-enhancer for many tubbers. The heightening of your senses provides a new dimension in sensuality. Imagine being submerged to your chin in a barrelful of massaging bubbles: cool, fresh air blowing on your upturned face, viewing heaven's neon—literally a million stars!

Marijuana and the hot tub make a dynamic duo. You won't feel as dizzy as you might with alcohol, and you will enjoy the air and water much more. Just make sure you don't feel so luxurious that you fall asleep!

Then comes the Munchies. Visions of sugarplums dance in your head—and Mallowmars, potato chips, Oreo cookies.... Anticipate those cravings and take a tray of assorted cheeses, iced grapes and crisp apple slices out to the deck with your wine. (We know your hot tub filter is good, but we don't think it'll do too well filtering a barrage of soggy potato chips or cookie crumbs, so mollify your tummy—and your filter—with easy to handle, less-messy munchies.)

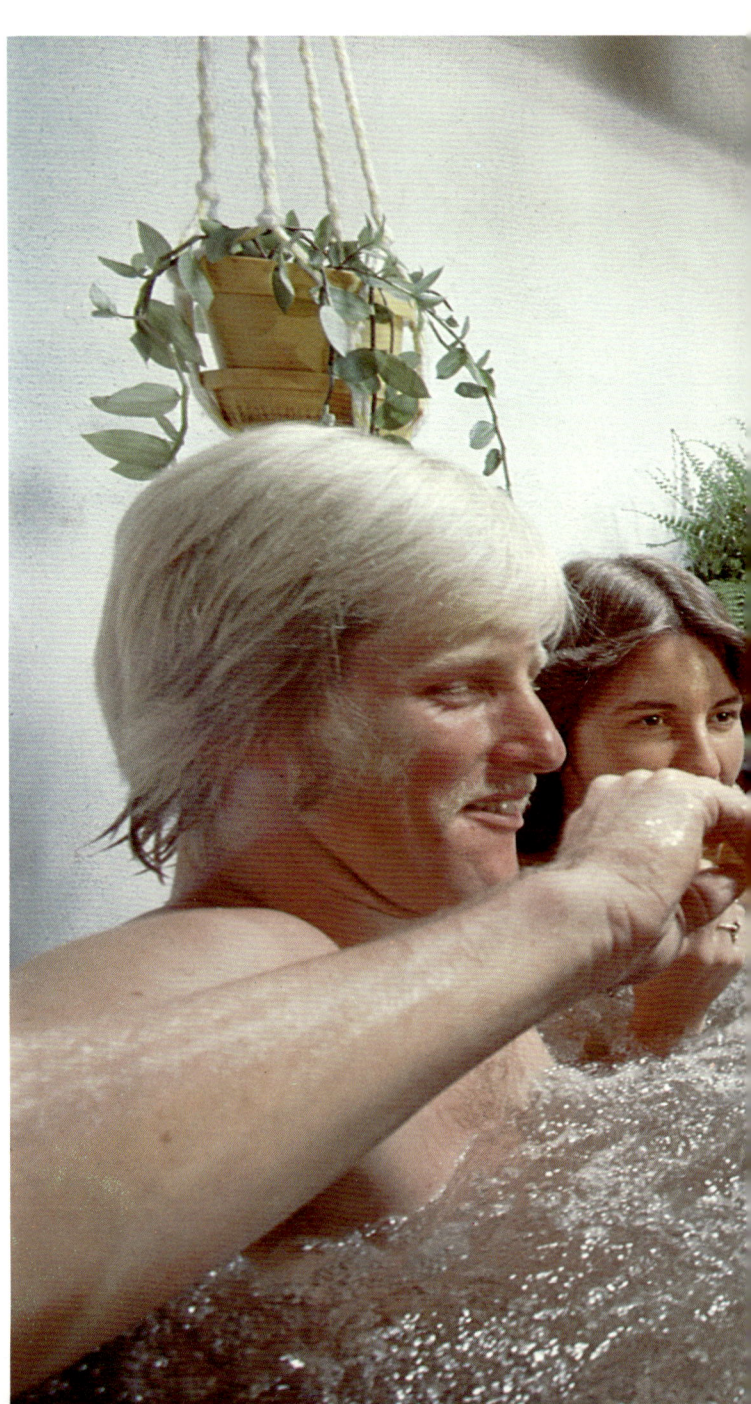

Munchies are within easy reach of all these hungry tubbers. The food-and-drink tray is on a simple rope-and-pulley system, which can be raised or lowered to any desired height. As people begin to fill the tub, the overflow of water normally lost is collected in the whiskey kegs in the background and is later piped back into the tub, still warm and ready to use again.

M-M-M-M-M-M-M-M-M-M

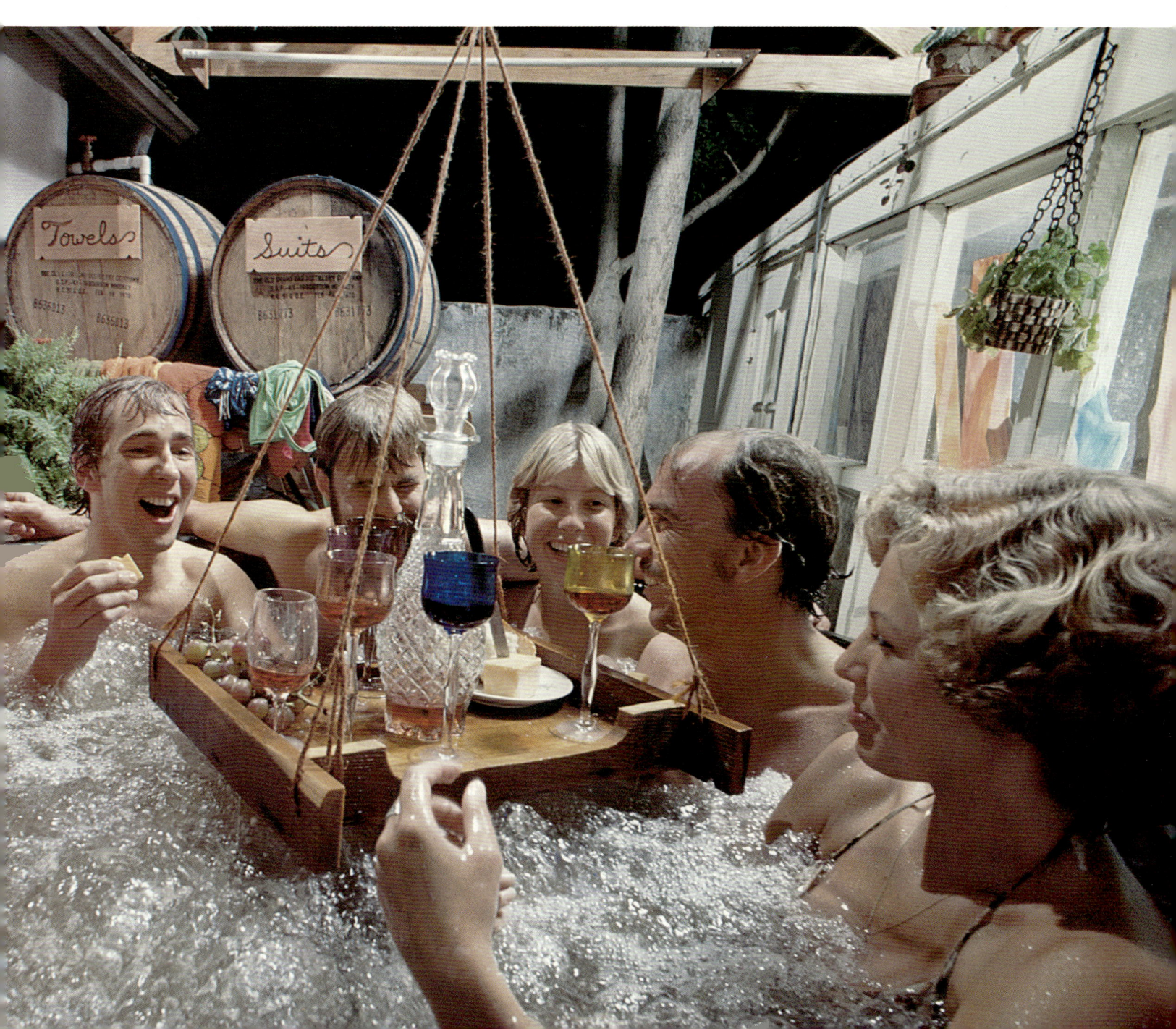

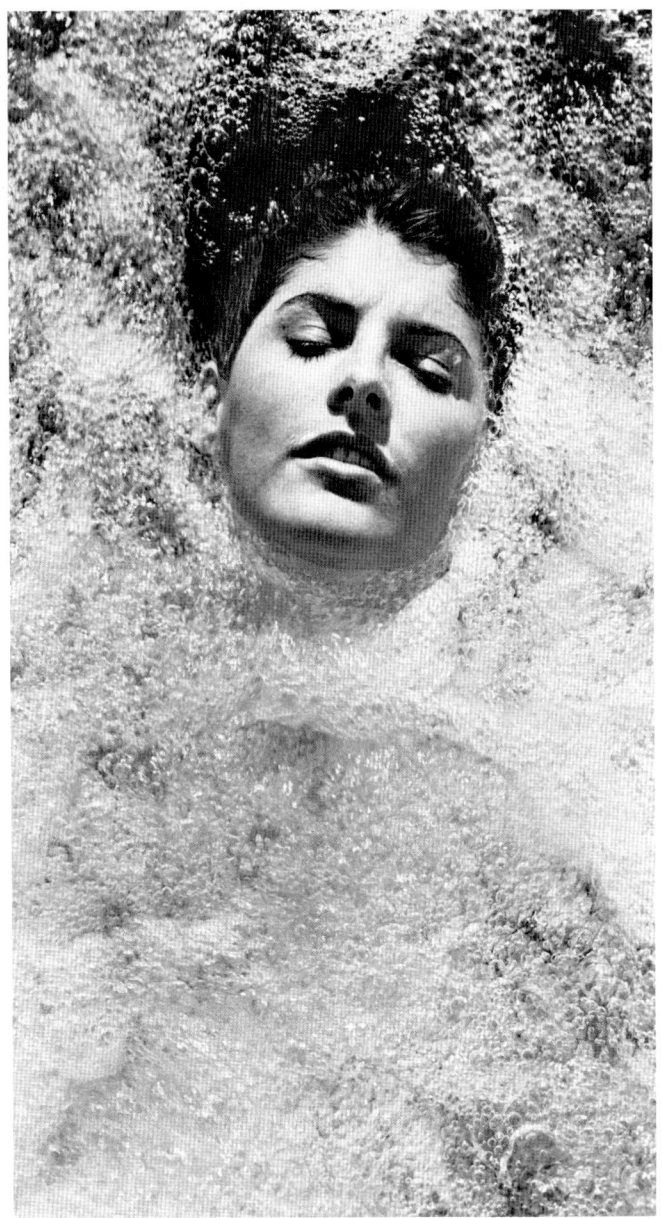

MEDITATION

The soothing, quasi-mystical atmosphere of your hot tub makes it an ideal spot to practice meditation. There's no need to take the phone off the hook, or to put a "DO NOT DISTURB" sign on your door. Just sit on a bench in your warm tub, close your eyes, listen to the birds sing and feel the warm sun on your face. Enjoy a relaxing twenty minutes with yourself and your own hum or mantra.

If you haven't yet met a guru and been presented with your own mantra for meditation, we have a treat for you. We asked Maharajah Maharani Mah-Jongg for a special hot-tub mantra. After *much* meditation, he disclosed a mantra to help you meditate in your hot tub. So listen closely, and don't tell anyone—here is your very own special hot-tub mantra: TSHOBUT.*

You can also practice yoga stretching and limbering exercises in the weightlessness of your tub. We don't recommend practicing the lotus position, or you'll spend half your time toppling off the bench into the water, and some of the more complicated positions could result in drowning, which might put an abrupt end to your meditative state. Peace.

*Hot Tubs scrambled.

Alone with your thoughts in warm surroundings and free from the restraints of clothing, the act of meditating becomes a sensual experience: to reflect; plan; achieve.

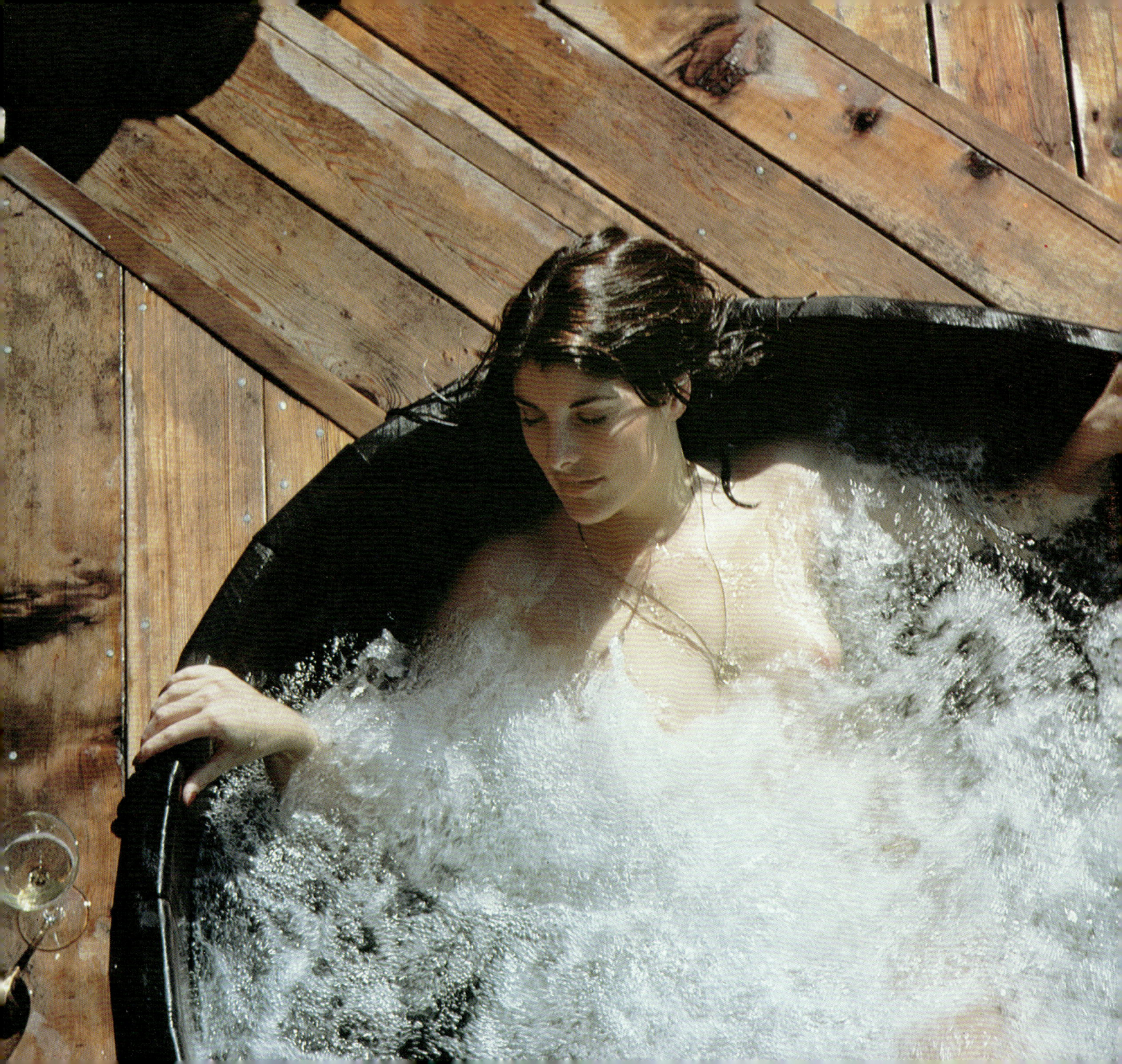

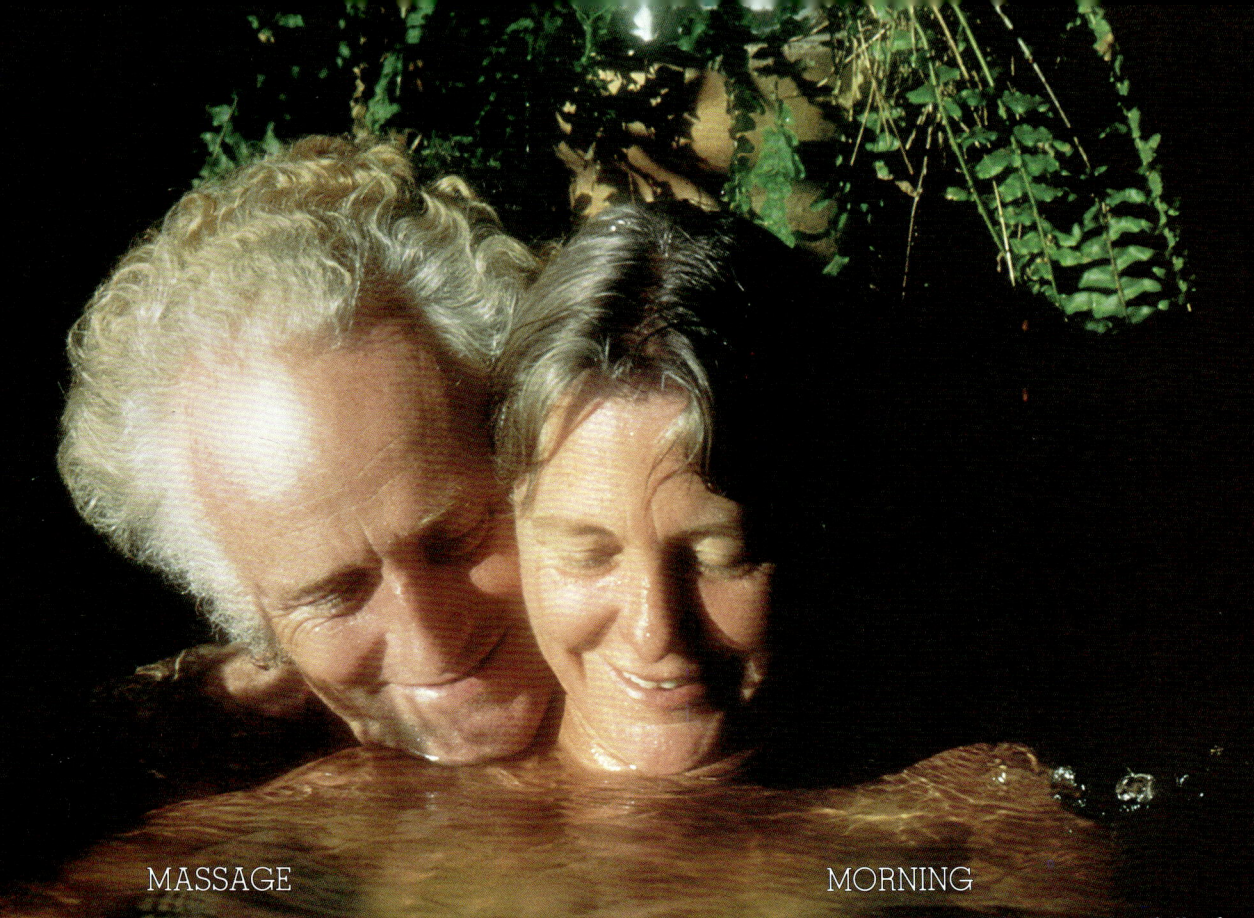

MASSAGE

A massage is a joy for those of us who enjoy being touched and the state of the art has thankfully come a long way from the famous "Mazola Oil" parties. There are many good massaging oils and essences available today. Some oils evaporate quickly; some are long-lasting and some are scented. All enhance the tactile, slippery delights of massage.

You can add a drop or two of the scented essences to your tub, but we recommend that if you use a liberal hand with the massaging oil, rinse off before climbing into your tub. The filter is good, but a frequent oil slick on your water doesn't help any. If you do use oils and your water gets messy, just allow the filtering system to run longer than usual until the water is clear again.

MORNING

Are you a lark, or a night owl? The world is full of morning people and night people. If you are a morning lark, you may enjoy hot tubbing best in the early hours while the rest of the owls are still snoozing off last night's revelry. If Henry David Thoreau had owned a hot tub, he would have marveled in early-morning tubbing.

Morning tubbing is an invigorating and happy way to wake up. Forget your usual shower—just slip out of bed and into your hot tub and let the tingling jets of warm water wake your body up. Relax and soak in your quiet time, and then go make your coffee. M-M-M-M-M-M-M-Merry, mirthful men and women, well-satisfied, well-rounded marvelous huManity.

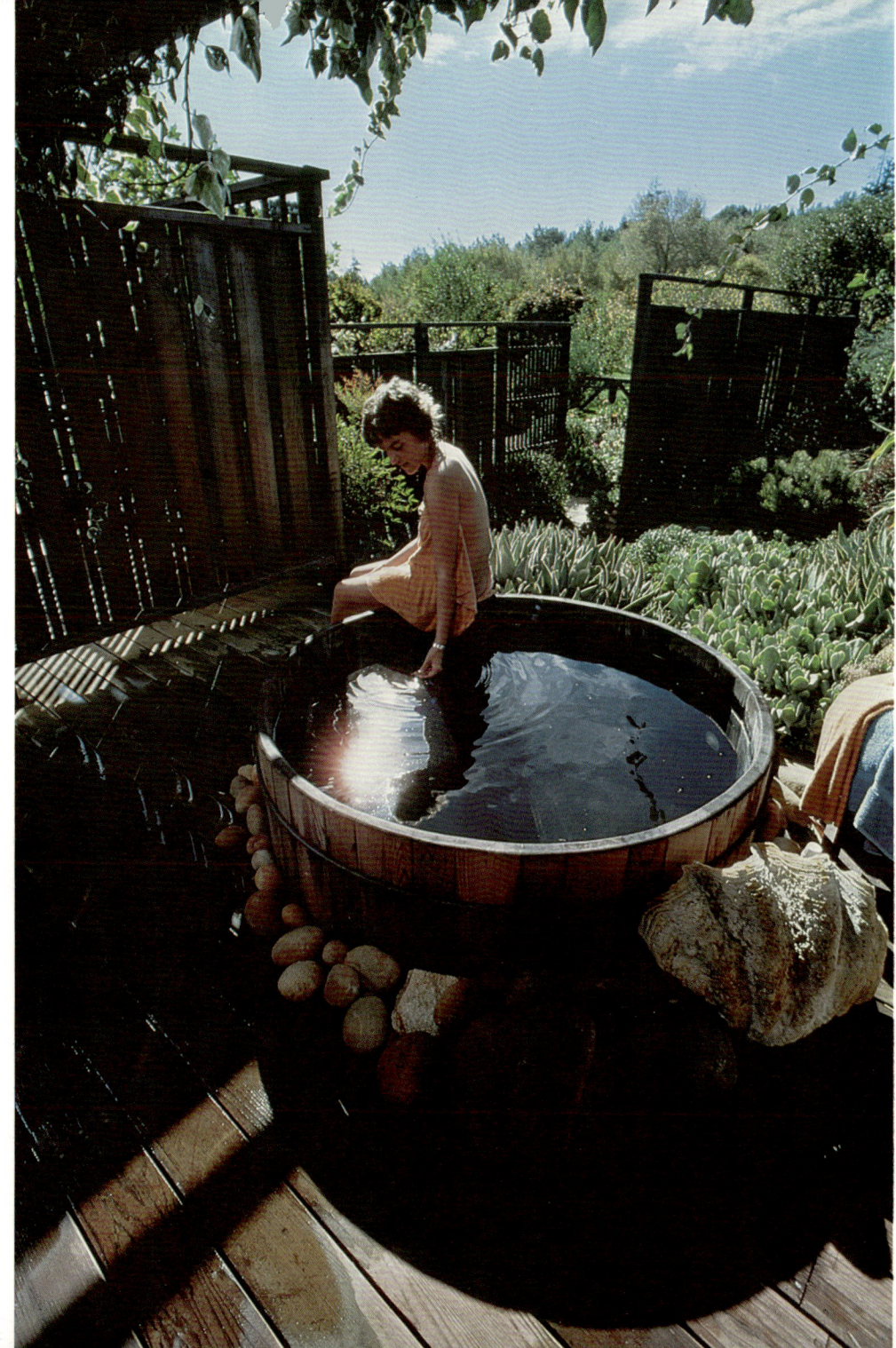

A formal garden provides a serene setting for an early-morning tubber. Rocks and shells surrounding the tub were obtained from a nearby riverbed and camouflage the above-deck plumbing.

CANNIBAL SOUP

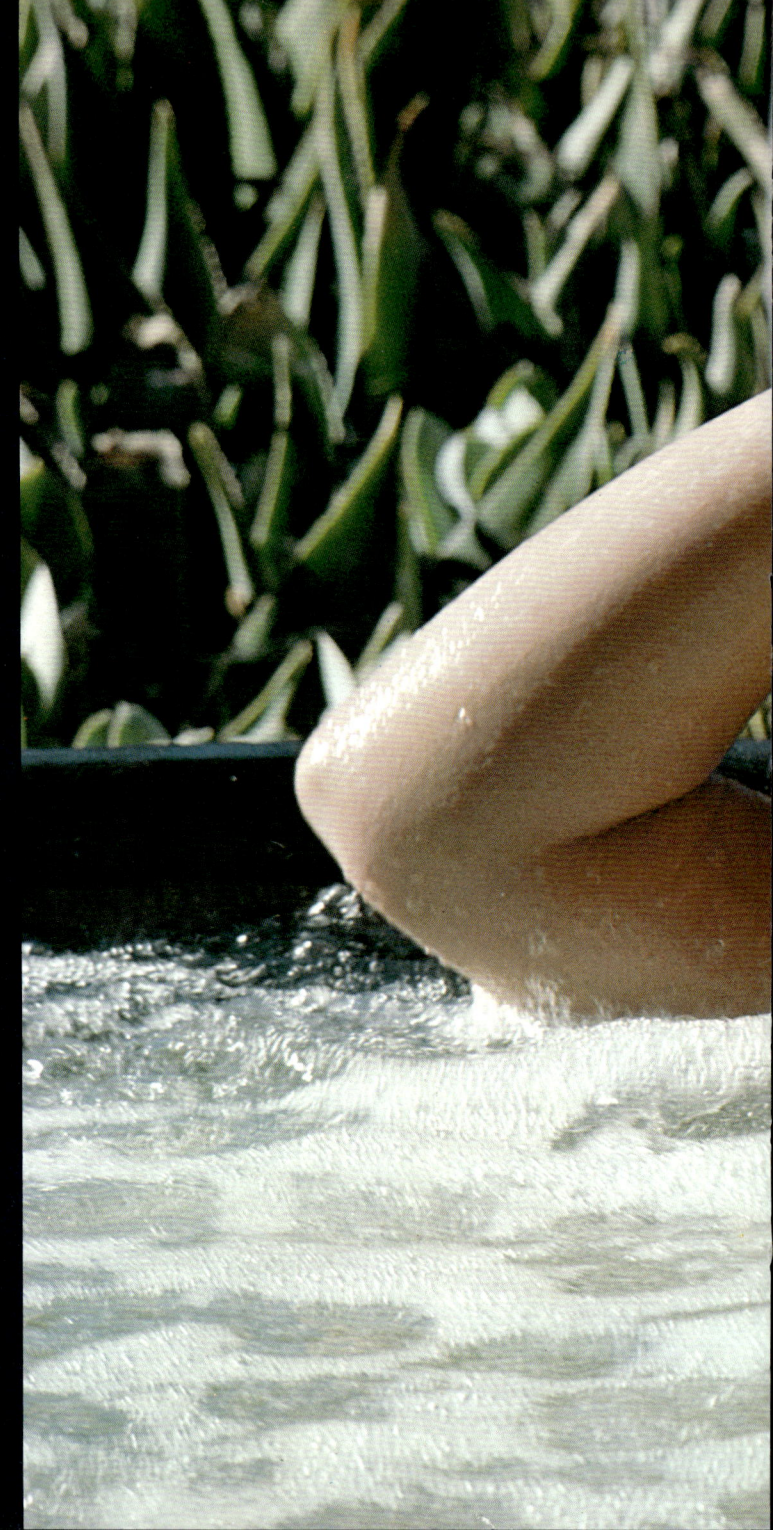

I have been as sincere a worshipper of Aurora as the Greeks. I got up early and bathed in the pond; that was a religious exercise, and one of the best things which I did. . . . The morning, which is the most memorable season of the day, is the awakening hour. Then there is least somnolence in us, and for an hour, at least, some part of us awakes which slumbers all the rest of the day and night. . . .

Thoreau—*Walden*

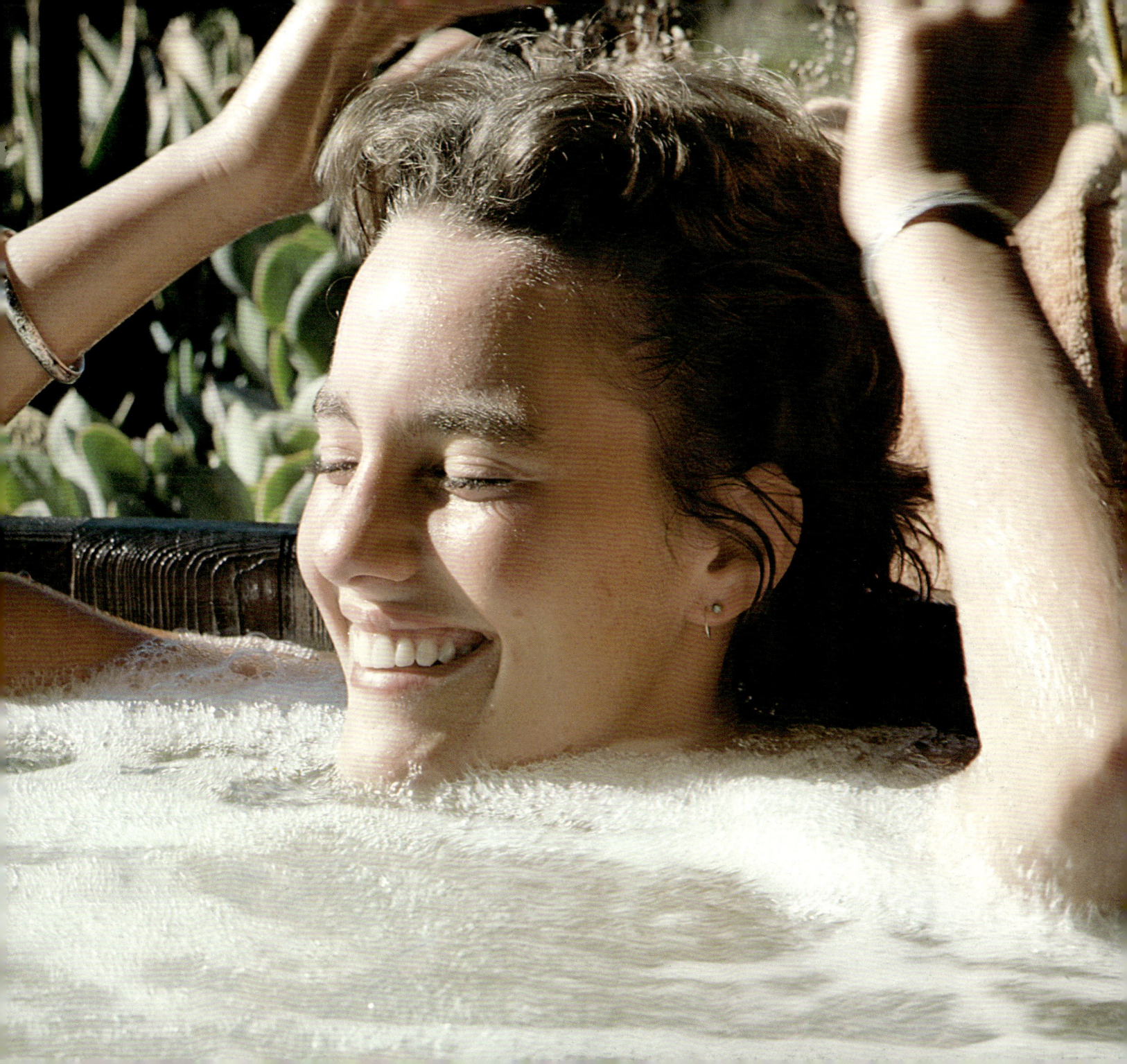

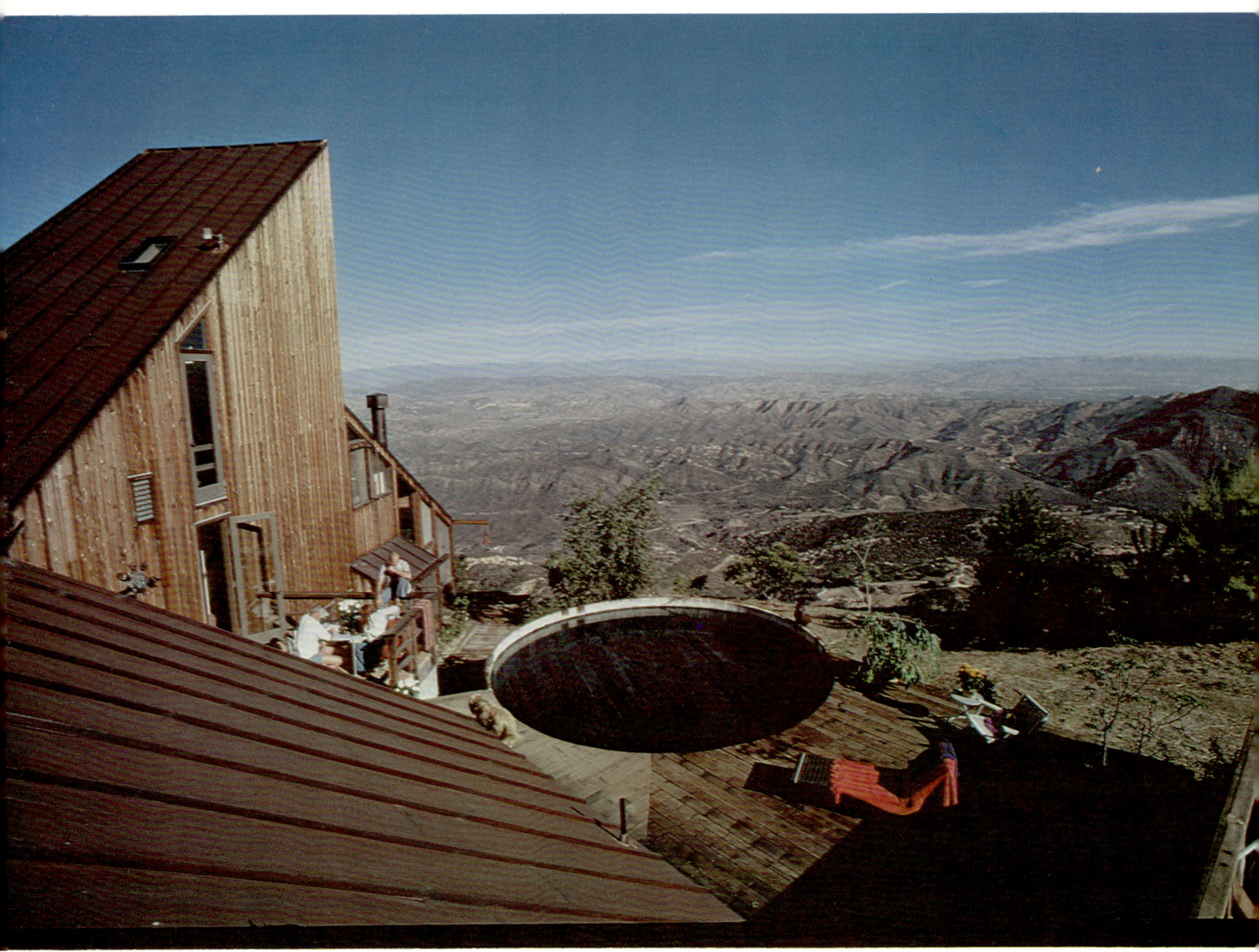

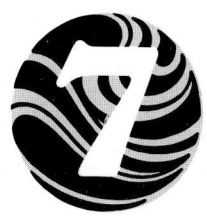

IF YOU'VE SEEN ONE, HAVE YOU SEEN THEM ALL?

In your search for the *right* hot tub you'll find that they come in as many shapes and sizes as the human body . . . almost. We've never seen a really ugly tub, but that's not to say that one couldn't be made. The tubs on the market are all called "hot tubs," but that's where the similarity ends. There are tubs made of redwood; of plywood coated with resin; of plastic; and of tile and coping like a traditional swimming pool. Many hot tubs have even been made out of old wine barrels or vats, which no doubt provides the owner with an additional treat to his sense of smell!

A tub can come in a variety of shapes and sizes. The most popular is a round tub called the barrel; the second most popular shape is the square tub. Sizes vary greatly. The smallest, the cuddle tub, is usually three feet wide and three feet deep. It holds two *very* good friends. Next, is the family-sized five feet across and four feet deep, and then come the larger six-by-four or six-by-five feet. The largest tub we've seen was a twenty-foot tub that was five feet deep and resembled a small lake.

A few points to consider when choosing the size and shape of your tub are: *Where will you put it? How big is your backyard or patio? How many people will use it?* Remember, the hot tub's togetherness factor. If there are four in your family you'll want a hot tub large enough to hold them comfortably. If you entertain a lot, perhaps you'll want a larger model to accommodate more people. *What size and shape will best fit into your environment?* Remember, some tubs are indoors.

The pictures in this book should give you some idea of which size and shape would best suit your needs. Let's now take a closer look at the materials that you might consider.

Redwood is the most beloved and widely used material. All redwood tubs are made from clear-heart redwood and they are moisture proof, and resistant to mildew and wood rot. Redwood is also

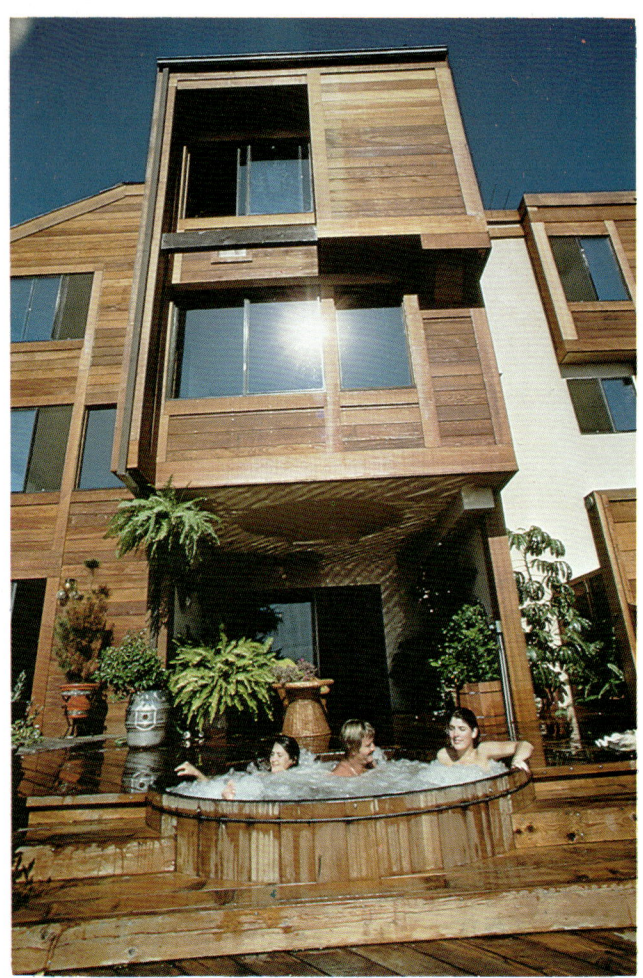

These two oval tubs crafted by Gordon and Grant of Santa Barbara, California, with creative deck design by Rex Marchbanks, add that touch of class to the already luxurious surroundings.

pleasant to the senses: sight, smell and touch. And, since the redwood tree is one of our oldest living things, sitting in that nice warm vat made of wood that is centuries old connects you to the past and to nature.

Some tub makers use plywood coated with resin and then surround the tub with a redwood skirting. Others use a plastic liner in a redwood frame. To each his own but either plastic or resin gives us the *bathtub* feel when we touch it, so we wholeheartedly chose *all* redwood. Tile and coping spas sunk into the ground fit well with a swimming pool that is already installed and some owners prefer them because they better suit their aesthetics.

The redwood tub, whether it's the cuddle tub or the jumbo family size, can be set up on your cement patio or on a prepared spot in your backyard in just a day or two. Then you can surround it with steps and decking to suit your personal taste, as we will discuss later. If you are interested in a *condo tub*—one which can be set up in the small area afforded by a patio or in the enclosed garage of your condominium or apartment—this can be arranged. If you have need of a special size or shape, most manufacturers will be glad to custom-make it for you. It will be more expensive, but most dealers are only too happy to oblige.

However, if you're a do-it-yourselfer, with a good set of tools, and an affinity for woodworking, you *can* make your own hot tub. Craig Yost, of Sacramento, California, went to his local lumberyard and bought clear-heart, vertical grain redwood. He milled the staves on a jointer, cut his own chime joists, dadoed and fit the bottom to the staves, much in the same manner that a cooper would. The result?

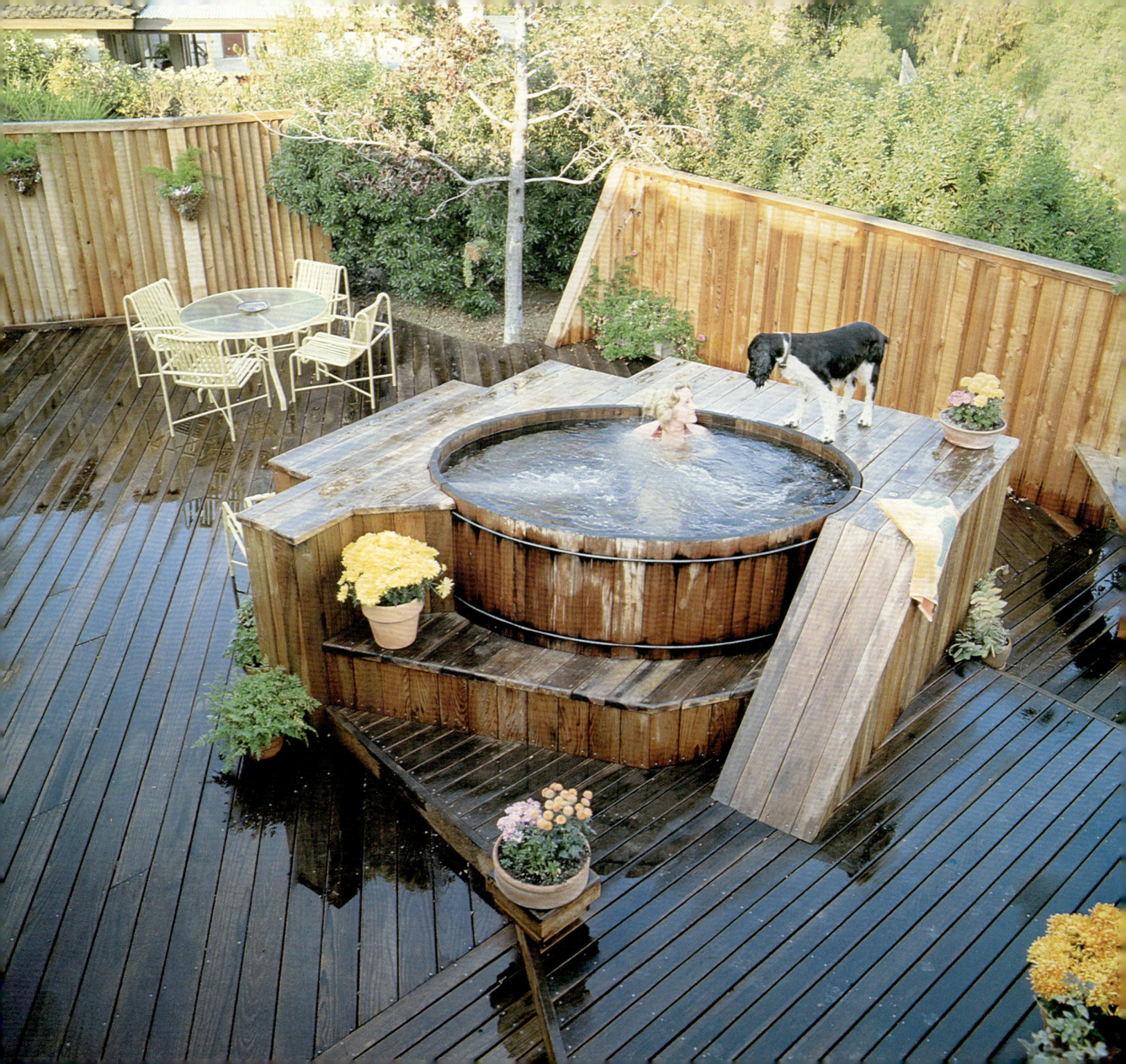

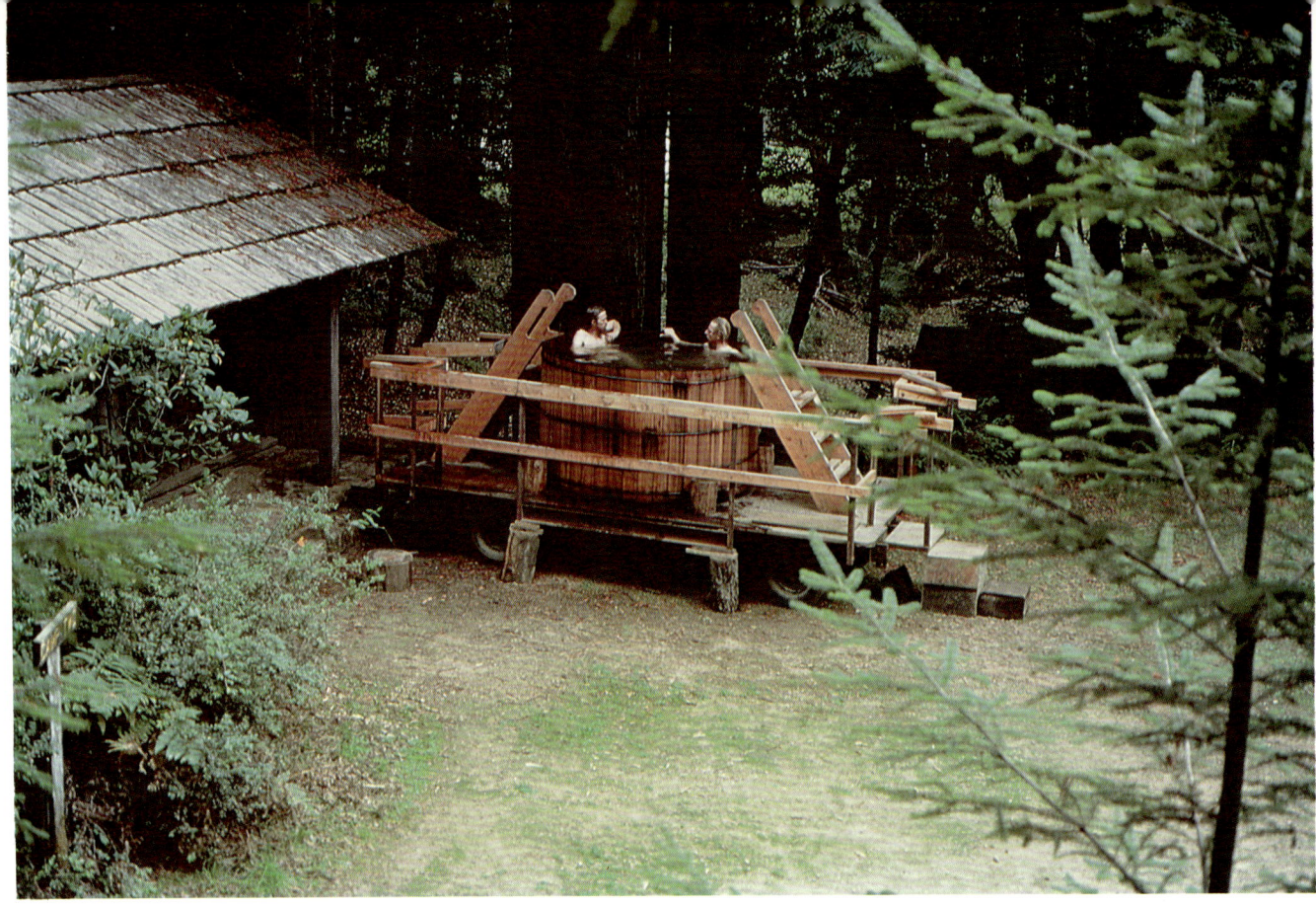

A fine-looking, five-foot-diameter tub with just that special touch of craftsmanship and individualism that sets it apart from a dealer tub.

Craig, an industrial arts teacher in a local high school, plans to incorporate the art of tub-making into his woodworking class; the students are already receiving orders! They plan to use the small profit from the project to purchase more tools and equipment for the high school shop.

So, with a bit of know-how, a little help from your friends, and some good equipment, you *can* make your own hot tub. You will, however, still have to invest in a commercial filter-pump-heater package for your tub, but your total cost will be about a third of the price of buying the tub ready-made. Most dealers are not set up to help the do-it-yourselfer; however, Spring Mountain Hot Tubs in Berkeley are most accommodating in providing detailed information which is very helpful to the amateur builder.

If you plan to set your tub outdoors, take into consideration the trees and shrubbery which will surround your tub. Your landscaping is important not only in creating the feeling you want—tropical

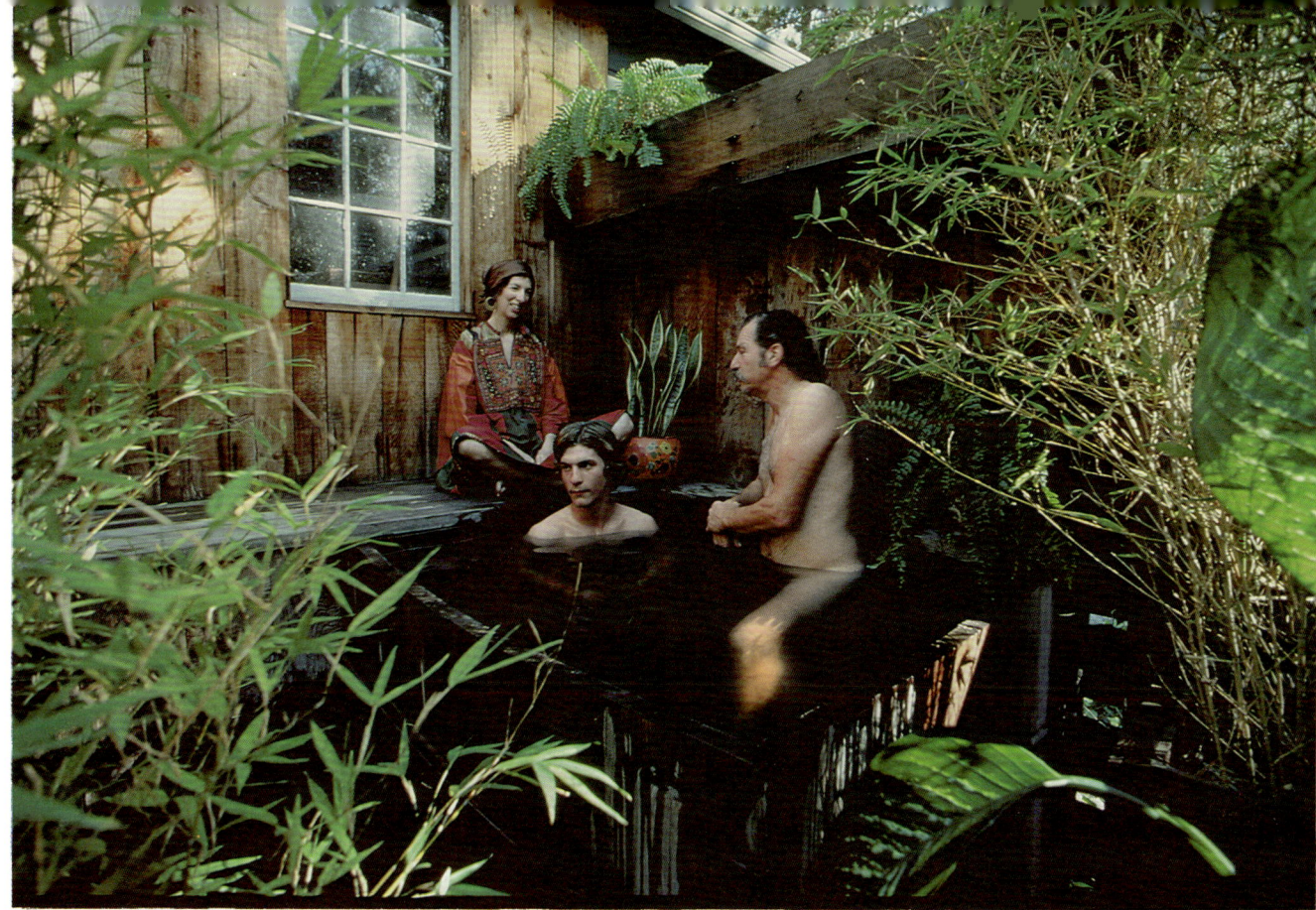

paradise or fern dell—but to give you privacy as well. In this age of tract homes and row upon row of closeness this last factor should be given *serious* consideration lest your neighbors forsake their nightly TV viewing for their nightly viewing *you*.

If you're as fortunate as we are, your tub will fit in among your present greenery. Our first tub was screened behind a bushy avocado tree, and when we simply placed a few potted plants and ferns around the decking the landscaping was complete. By the way, ferns and other hanging plants do very well in the moist steamy atmosphere of a hot tub. Do try to locate your tub away from "dirty" trees however, or you'll be skimming off a lot of leaves and bird droppings before you can climb into your tub.

The mobile hot tub on the left was created by the Mendocino Woodlands Camp for use by its campers. Tub, pump and heater are all mounted on a flat-bed truck and driven to sites as needed. The handmade square tub, pictured above, is used as a unique karate exercise arena for the owners' son. The bamboo provides a natural privacy shield for all.

LIGHTS! MUSIC!

Now let's look at the finishing touches. Nothing adds more to your enjoyment of a hot tub than listening to your favorite music—a little Bach or Brahms with your bubbles, maybe? Many people extend speakers outside from their in-house stereo, and some "sound freaks" have a complete component system installed near the tub. This is fine, but remember, those units use electricity, and you are going to be wet. . . . If piped-in music is not feasible, open a nearby window and turn up the volume of your

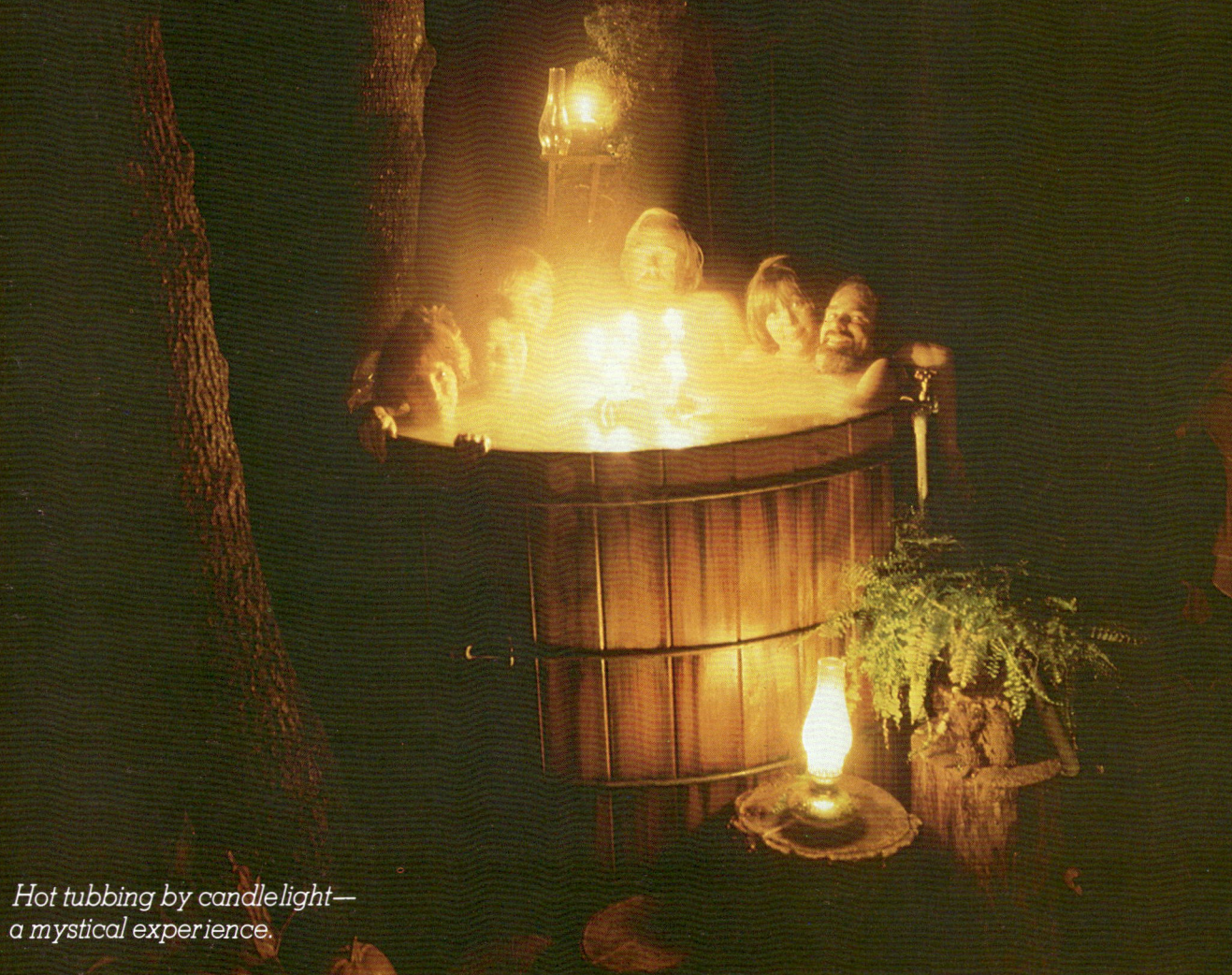

*Hot tubbing by candlelight—
a mystical experience.*

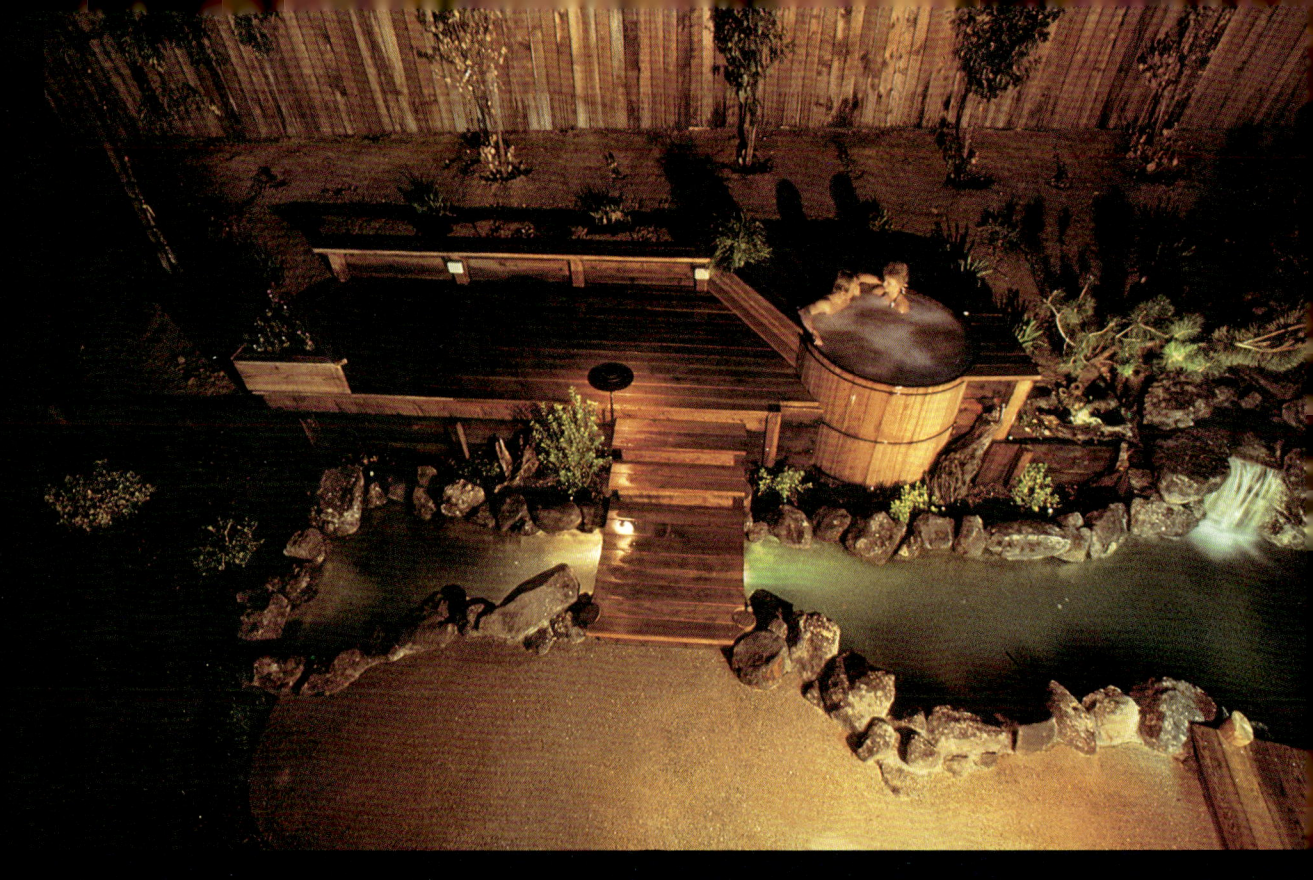

radio or stereo. The only drawback is that when the air jets are turned on, the music is tuned out.

We also have found a little indirect lighting near the steps of our decking is a valuable aid for navigation by night to and from the tub, but too much illumination spoils the effect of the moonlight shining down through the trees. So use a little artfully. One owner, whose tub was located on his patio, used indirect lighting on the shrubs around the perimeter of his yard and created a soft green curtain of color. Since we so love astronomy we prefer very muted light around our tub in so as to not inhibit our gazing at heavenly bodies. Try placing a few candles around your deck area; candlelight and moonlight are the most flattering and romantic lighting for those quiet evenings anyway.

mentioning price. To ask how much a hot tub costs is like asking the cost of an automobile. It depends on size, equipment and other options. Also, some dealers run specials on certain size tubs during the year, or throw in options as an inducement to buy. As a general rule, however, prices for a complete tub vary from one to ten thousand dollars for the more lavish models. Look for hot-tub dealers in the home-improvement section of your favorite magazine or newspaper, or the Yellow Pages of your telephone book. Any hot-tub dealer can give you a price breakdown in accordance with what you need. Some hot-tub companies will even arrange to loan you a demonstration tub for a weekend while you explore the delights of a hot bubbling spa right in your own backyard. Let them show you their

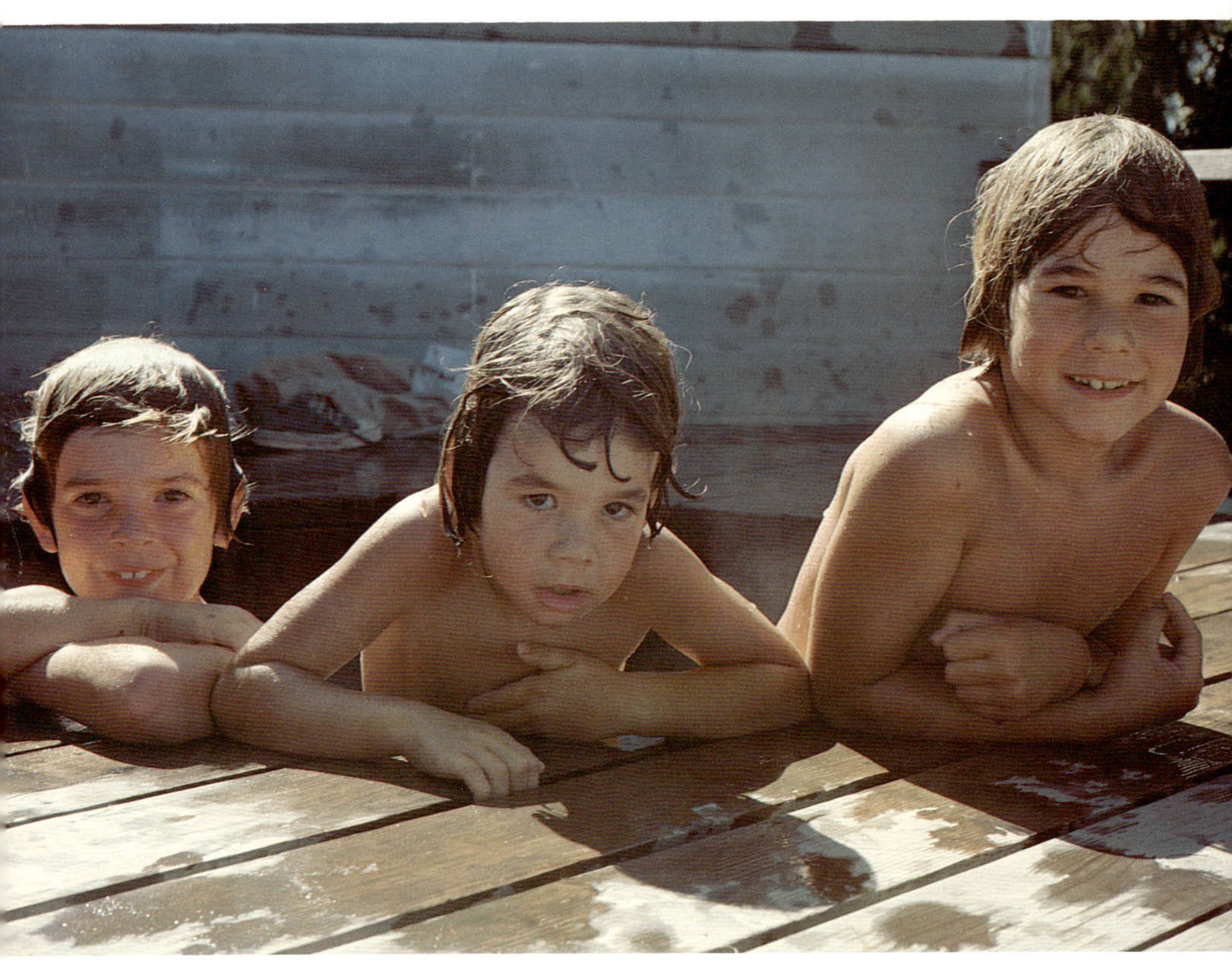

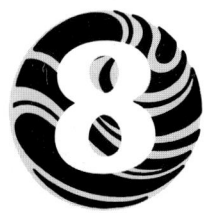

TO DECK OR NOT TO DECK?

No matter what size hot tub you choose, you'll need some sort of platform or deck around it to make getting in and out of it easier and safer and to have a place to put your wine glasses. The first few weeks we had our tub, we used a stepladder and a picnic table while we gathered material to do our decking. This was a rather ingenious temporary deck—we thought—until one night Valerie's mother stepped on the edge of the wet table. It tipped, and Mother and stepladder did a joint swan dive onto the patio. Fortunately, she bruised only her dignity but the next day our deck construction did begin in earnest. We were fortunate also that the swan-diver wasn't Sue Happy Sue from down the street instead. Such an accident might have given her a very luxurious trip to the French Riviera—to recuperate.

So decking is important for both safety and appearance and if you must use your tub the first few days with temporary decking, be sure that it's safe. Wet feet and a wet rickety ladder could mean a bad injury.

Most hot tub dealers also build and install decking. Decking is an option and like all options, the more you want, the more it costs. All decking installed by your dealer is of quality redwood, just like your tub, and usually consists of four-by-four posts, two-by-fours for framing and two-by-sixes for surface material. All posts are sunk in concrete; latticework and trim can be added as you desire.

You should keep in mind that a dealer-built deck—although more expensive than the deck you build yourself—will be a deck custom-fitted to your tub by men who do this job every day. There is nothing like having the job done by an expert. But, if you are on a limited budget, or if you have had some prior experience at building, then there is a less expensive way to go.

We found custom decking a little too much for our pocketbook. A three-foot-wide deck around our tub with one ladder approach listed for $350. We wanted a deck four feet wide to start at our bedroom door, run halfway around the house, surround the tub and end at our family room door. We also wanted three different step approaches: one from the garden; one from the backyard; and one near the tub itself. It was obvious the only way to achieve all this and still be able to eat was to build it ourselves.

Building a deck is like building any kind of structure—the important thing is to *do it right*; otherwise it will constantly disappoint you. Look over your site; consider the bushes and trees already there. It may be better to build your deck around an existing tree rather than remove the tree and discover later you have removed a portion of your natural privacy and have to plant something new in its place. So draw up a sketch of what you plan to build. If you aren't good at sketching, perhaps an artist or draftsman friend can help. A few well-thought-out plans can save you time and material as well.

Because your deck is a conspicuous addition to your house, the material you use deserves thoughtful attention also. You will be selecting material for three main parts of your deck: the surface; the supporting framework and the foundation. You can choose from among many different kinds of materials for surface and support but the choice for the foundation is a limited one—concrete. In your choice for surface and supporting material you can use either new or used lumber, but remember, you want something which will withstand moisture well.

We built our deck out of used redwood lumber. We are blessed with a used lumberyard in our town that is not only a browser's paradise, but a source of great bargains as well. We built 380 square feet of deck as described earlier, using two-by-eights for

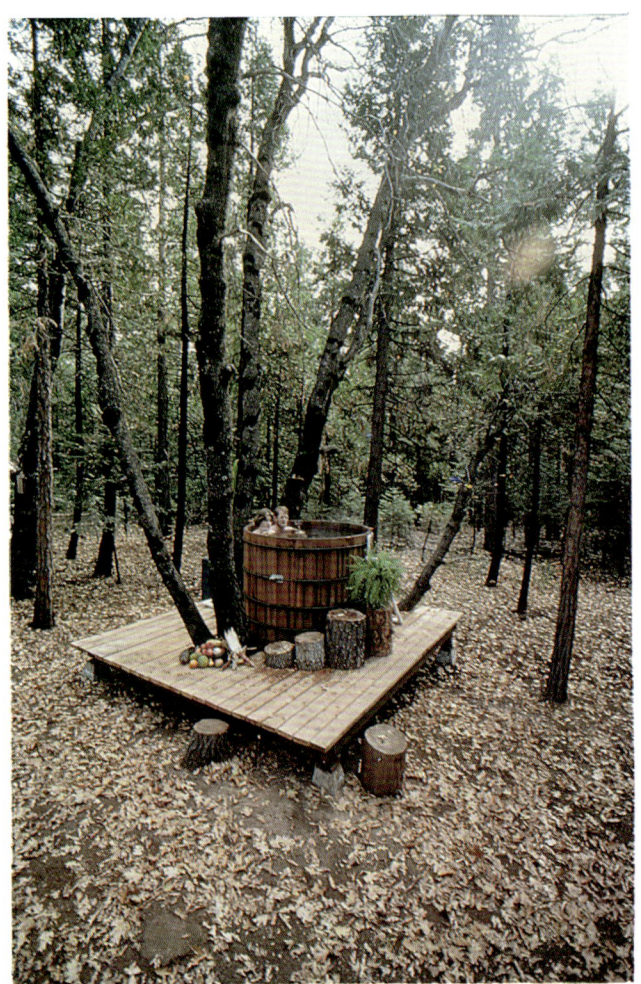

Simple, but effective—the deck above was built around existing trees, to avoid disrupting its natural surroundings. The tubs on the right double your pleasure—a cold tub on the top and a hot tub on the bottom.

To Deck or Not to Deck?

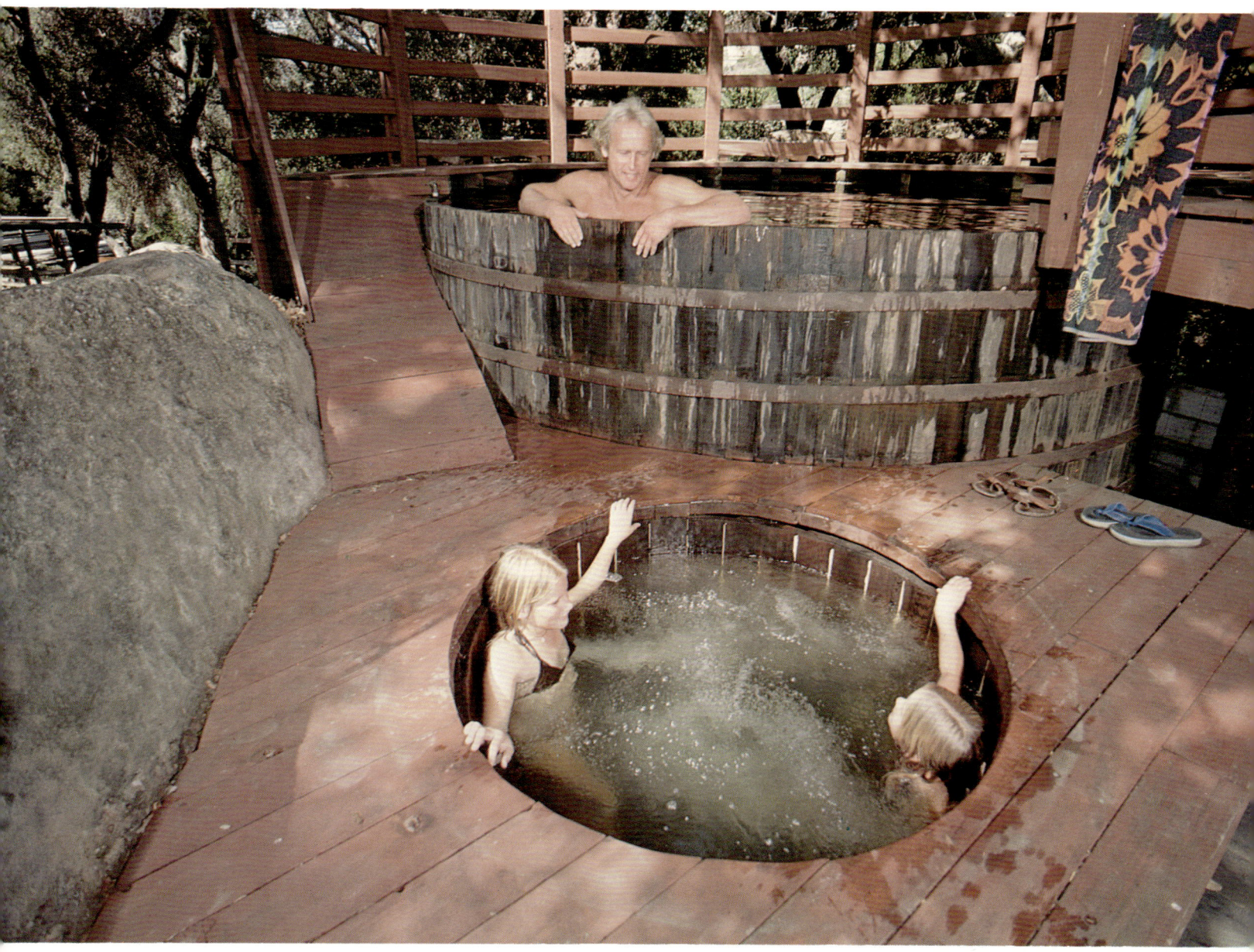

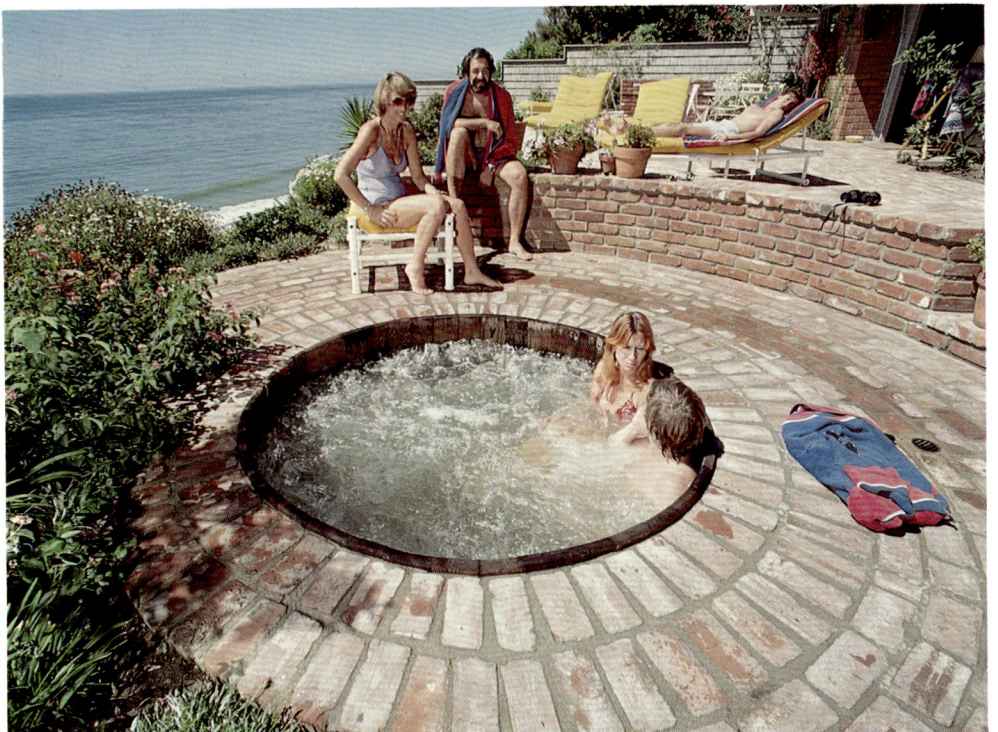

Decks don't have to be made of wood. Here, brick laid in a radiating pattern accents the roundness of the tub. Similar designs can be achieved by use of cobblestone or flagstone. Let your own imagination work for you.

surface lumber, two-by-sixes and four-by-fours for the supporting framework. Total cost: four hundred dollars. Naturally, we could have used new lumber and still have made substantial savings, but as we said, our budget was limited and our decking needs were rather specialized, so used lumber filled our bill best. We had to contend with old nail holes and rough cuts, but with lots of sanding and a little wood filler, we covered the unwanted flaws, and found that the wood's rugged appearance added to the effect that we wanted.

Standard dimension lumber is most commonly used for surface material. These are: two-by-twos, two-by-threes, two-by-fours, two-by-sixes, and two-by-eights. We used two-by-eights—anything wider than a two-by-eight tends to "cup" or warp crosswise and make an uneven, scooped surface. We nailed the two-by-eights a half inch apart to allow for expansion and the ease of water runoff. Some decking instructions advise a width of a quarter inch to avoid stubbing small toes, but since we don't have the patter of tiny feet around our deck, we opted for the wider space.

The supporting framework below the deck's surface consists of joists, beams and posts. We used two-by-sixes for joists, two-by-fours for cross-

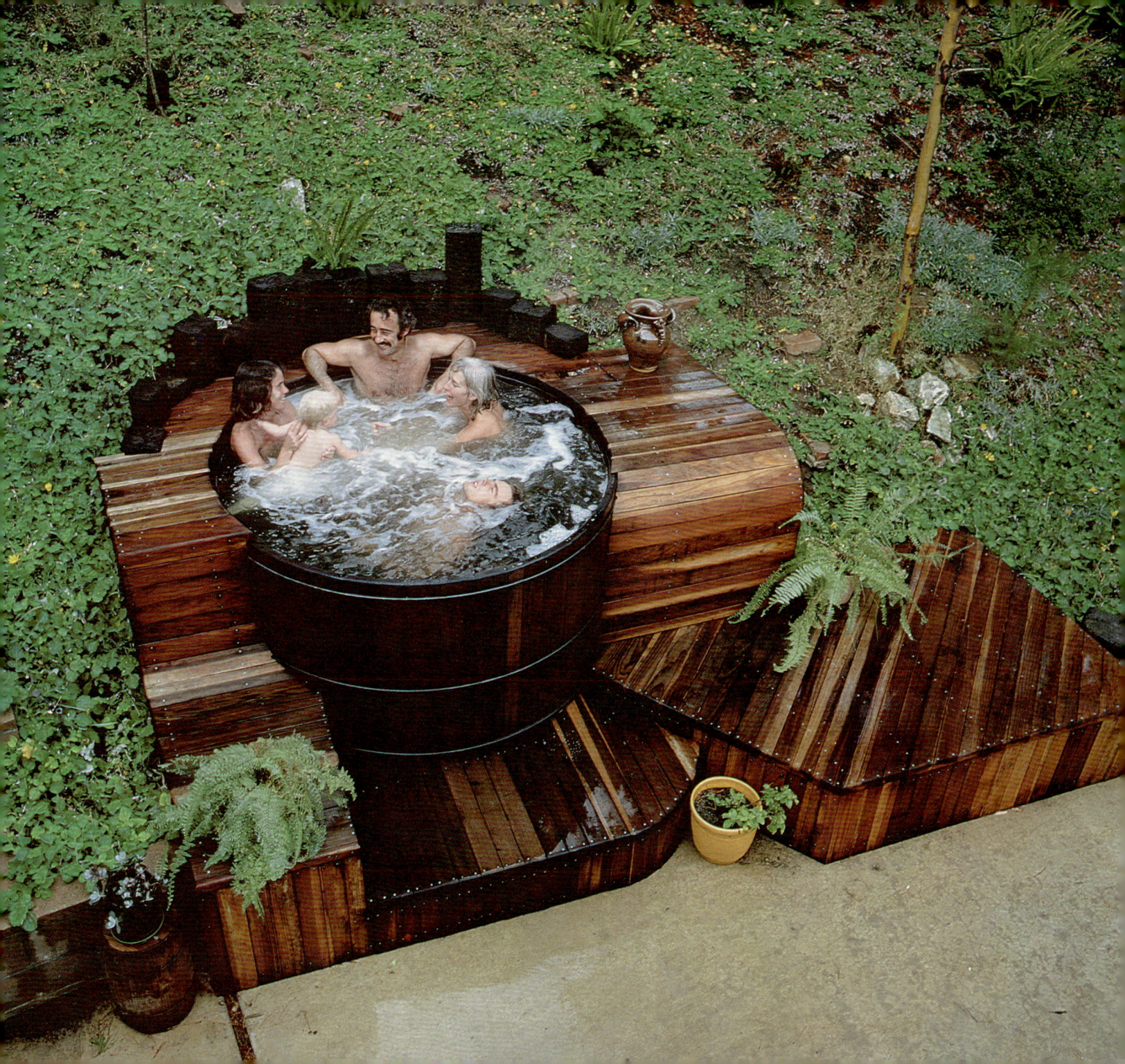

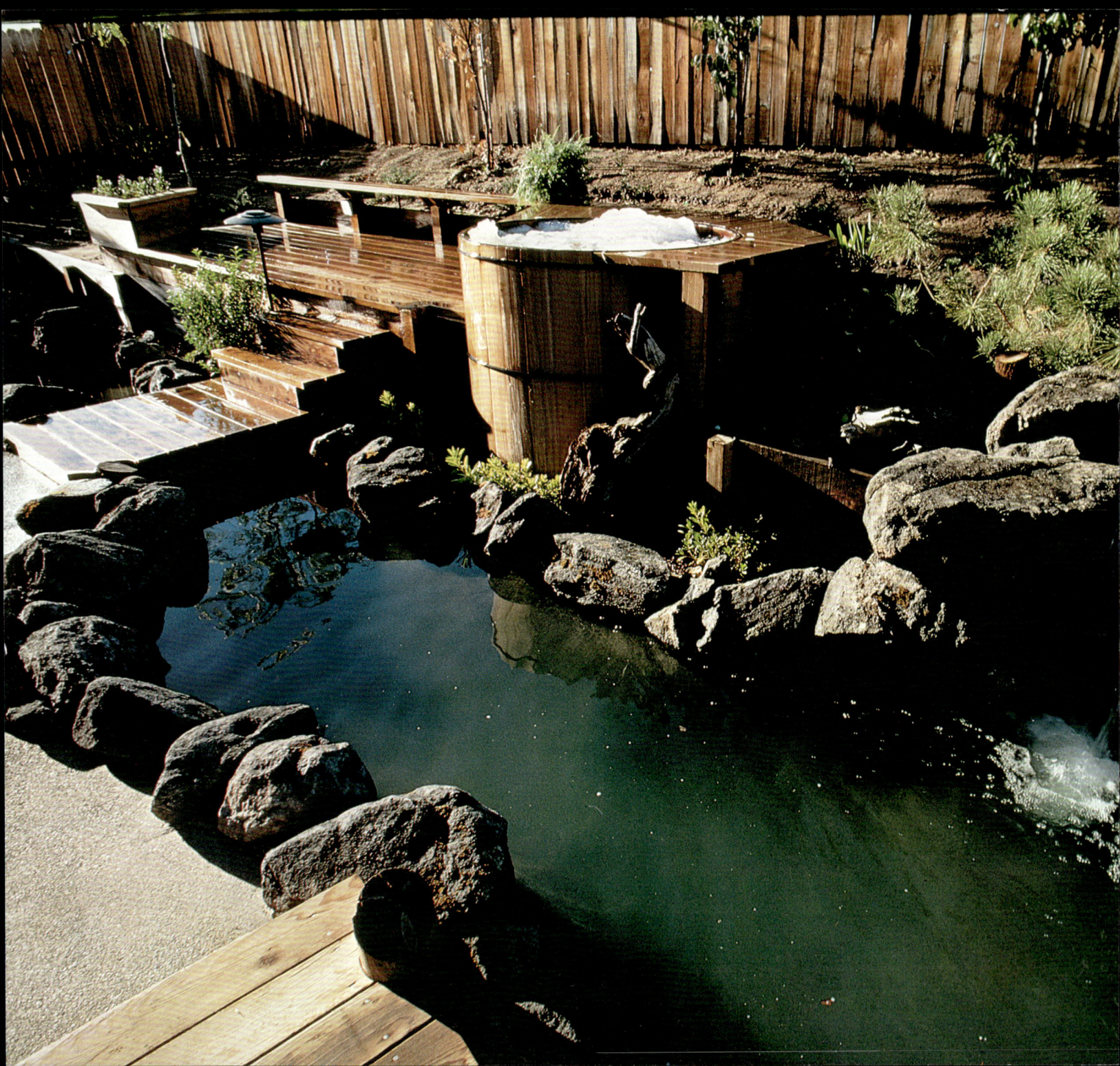

Zierden Landscaping of Sacramento, California, created this hot tub lagoon in a suburban backyard.

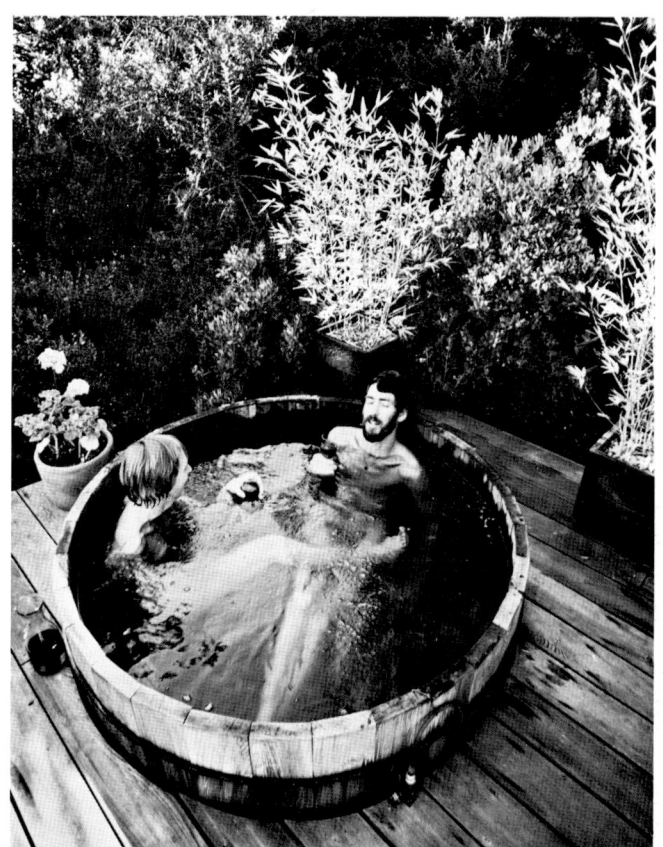

bracing, and four-by-fours for posts. One of the drawbacks of working with used lumber is the odd lengths the material comes in. We also found in some of our joist runs we needed a two-by-six longer than the standard lumber length of twenty-four feet. We solved both of these problems by sandwiching and splicing two pieces together to get the desired length. This is a simple method of butting two lengths of lumber together and sandwiching a three-foot piece on each side of the butt, then bolting and glueing the whole works together. We found that this was a way of putting the waste lumber to good use.

The posts—as mentioned before—were four-by-fours, cut to desired lengths and sunk into eighteen inches of concrete. Your concrete footings should extend at least six inches above ground to prevent moisture and/or termites from getting to the posts. *Check your local building codes on all conditions before you begin to build.* For example, some building codes won't allow posts set in concrete footings; only concrete piers can be used. It all depends upon what part of the country you live in and the rigidity of the building codes and restrictions. Wherever you are, and whatever the codes, adhere to them. They are usually for your protection, and remember, this deck is an addition to your home and must be up to code in order to sell.

You might prefer to seal and stain the surface of your deck. What you do will depend upon the weather conditions in your part of the country, and the type of wood you use. We found, with redwood or cedar, that linseed oil or a stain and sealer combined works well and gives an attractive appearance.

The last thing to consider is, whatever lighting you desire, remember to make all outlets and lighting waterproof. As mentioned before, a little lighting goes a long way. Let nature's moon and stars be your major light sources. What you add should be for safety and special effects.

Now, lie back in your hot tub and look out over your decking. Look at the spaciousness of it all; a lounging chair; a bench; a barbecue at one end; potted flowers here and there. The decking is an extension of your hot tub which unites it with the rest of your house. After you have warmed up in your tub, stretch out on your new deck and cool off as the water evaporates from your skin; nature's air-conditioning at work.

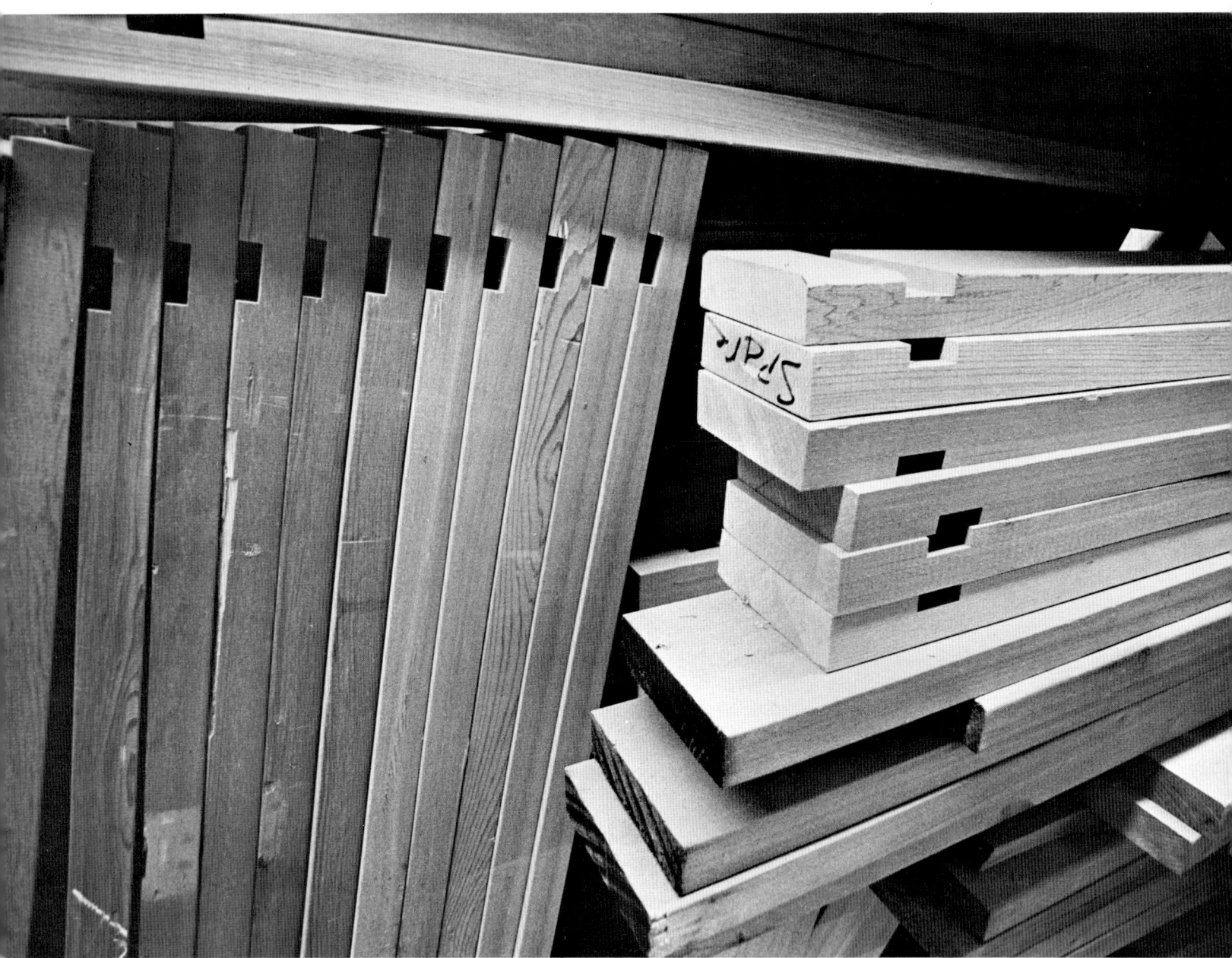

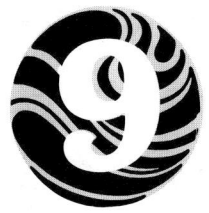

THE PARTS OF YOUR TUB NOBODY SEES

You've heard the old adage, "You get what you pay for..."? Never is it more true than in the purchase of a hot tub and its equipment. Don't buy your tub on the basis of price alone. You're not just buying another household appliance; you're adding a new dimension to your life. Permanently installed, it can be a substantial home improvement, or it could be moved to your new home if you move. In any case, your hot tub should give you years of pleasure.

The cooper takes great pains in selecting the wood which goes into your tub. A good tub begins with all-heart, straight-grained, thoroughly dried redwood. The tub walls are formed from slightly concave boards milled from two-inch stock; these are called staves. These staves fit together to produce a watertight container.

The floor supports, or chime joists, are notched to the tub and engineered to bear the weight. Hoops of steel are placed around the tub to help hold it together. These hoops are threaded on each end and lug nuts are used to tighten or loosen the hoops. Your tub will fit together easily without the use of nails or glue. After filling with water, the staves then swell to form a watertight fit.

No tub is any better than the quality of its equipment. The water must be heated, filtered and circulated through the system to the tub and back again. A centrifugal water pump driven by an electric motor circulates the water through both the filter and the heater. The pump contains a hair and lint trap which catches debris before it reaches the filter. This trap is easily cleaned by rinsing it with water.

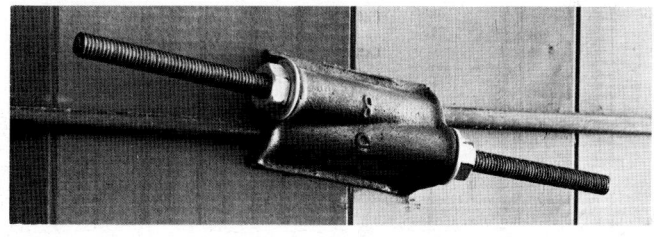

A double-lugged hoop—position away from traffic.

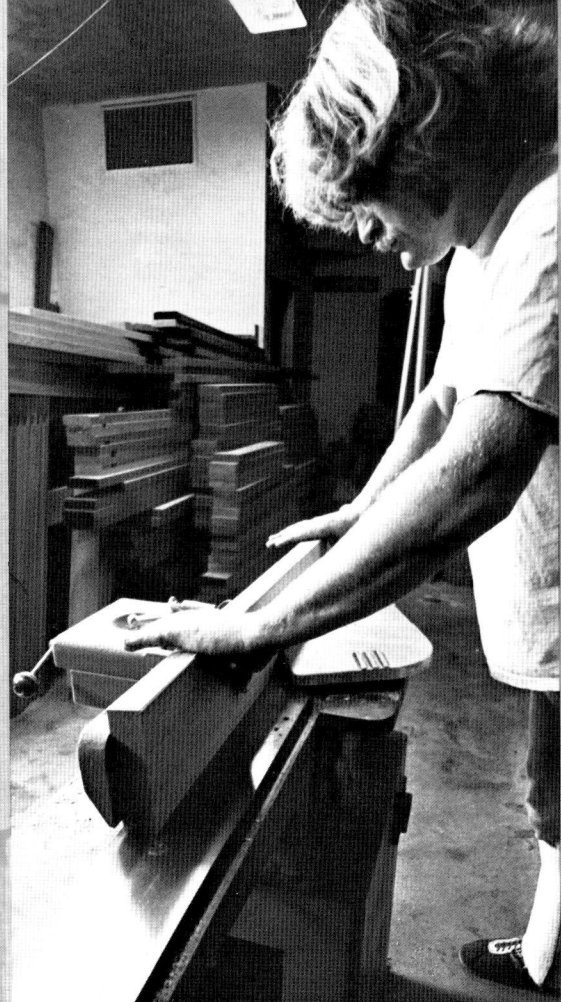
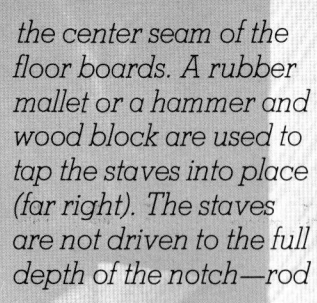

All heart, vertical-grained redwood is cut and milled smoothly for the staves. The staves (shown in the background) are notched to fit the bottom, and the edge of each stave is beveled slightly to fit snugly with the next one (far left). No nail or glue is used in the assembly. Four or more ½-inch steel hoops are tightened around the tub with single or double lugs, pressing each stave against the other. This, combined with the weight of the water and the natural swelling of the wood, creates a watertight tub. The bottom of the tub (second from left) is assembled with dowel pins with the rim beveled to fit the notched staves. The bottom is assembled with the beveled edges turned downward toward the ground (second from right). Three 4×4 redwood chime joists are placed under the floor at right angles to the floor boards. The weight of the tub rests on these chime joists—not on the staves—to prevent leakage. The first stave is placed so the center of the stave meets the center seam of the floor boards. A rubber mallet or a hammer and wood block are used to tap the staves into place (far right). The staves are not driven to the full depth of the notch—rod tightening will accomplish this later. Another stave is placed next to the first and tapped into place. The three strips of wood nailed to the bottom help hold the bottom together and are

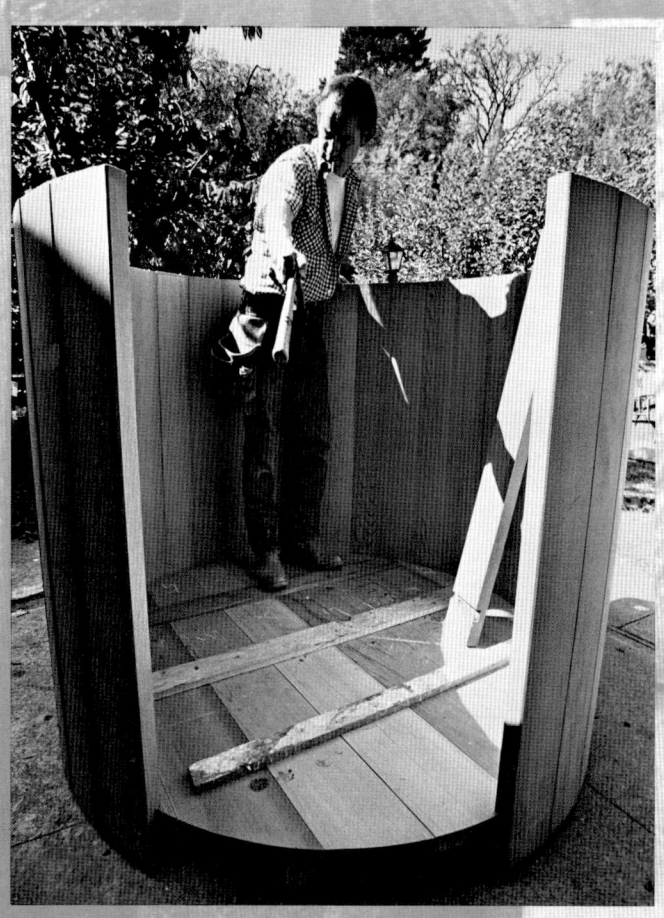 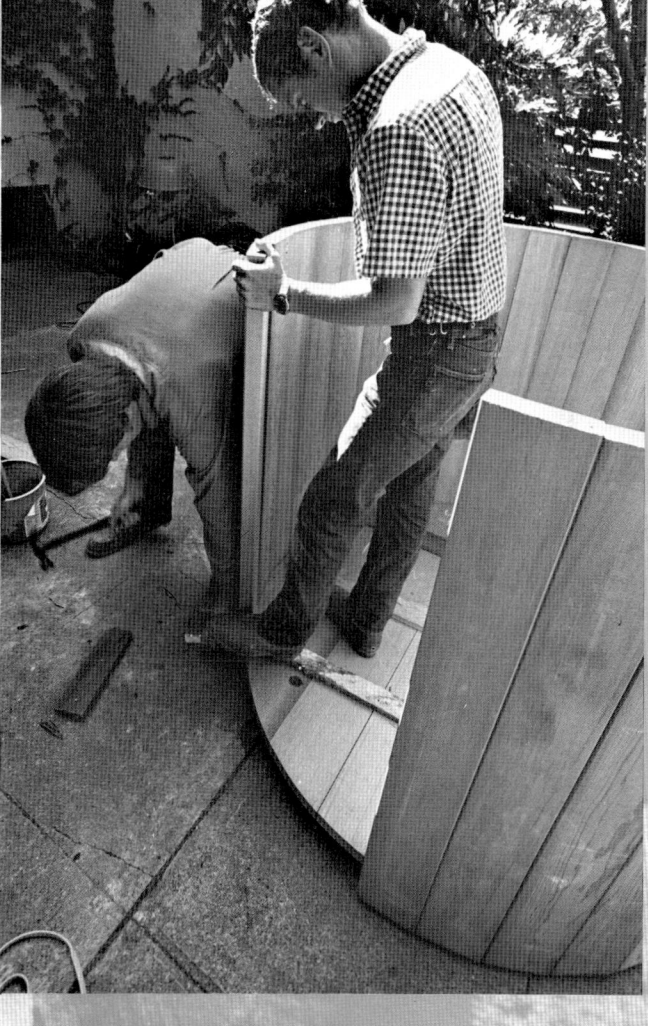

removed after the staves are all in place. Rods are then hung on temporary nails, and tightened until the lug is touching the wood. Each rod is tightened equally as a helper taps the staves on the inside until they are even at each point. This procedure is repeated until equal tension is achieved on each rod (overleaf). The benches are then installed and the holes drilled for the hydrojets. The jets are placed near each bench to provide a convenient back massage. The plumbing is then connected to the equipment and the tub's rim is sanded until smooth. The tub is now ready to be filled with water.

FILTERS & PUMPS

The type of filter is critical only in the fact that it should be large enough to keep the water in the system clean with a minimum of effort on your part. There are three types of filters: cartridge, permanent medium (sand and gravel) and diatomaceous earth. The diatomaceous earth and the cartridge type are removed and cleaned with water and tri-sodium-phosphate, while the permanent medium is backflushed to clean it. Your dealer can recommend which filter to use with your system. They all do the job, and it's really a matter of choice, which you and your dealer discuss.

Water is circulated through the system at approximately sixty gallons per minute using 1½-inch, noncorrosive PVC lines, so the size of your pump must be large enough to carry this load. The pump should have a bronze housing, which will eliminate warp and rust, and sealed bearings to eliminate oiling and to insure smooth running at high speeds. A ½- to 1-horse, 220-volt motor is used to drive the pump, and should be thermo-protected and well-grounded. The pump in the picture on the right has a built-in strainer basket to prevent hair, leaves and lint from entering. The heater in this system is gas and will not fire unless the pump is running, thus preventing the possibility of burning out the heating coils.

Some dealers use a convection heater in their systems. This type of heater relies on the process of convection—the natural tendency of hot water to rise. It is attached to the tub by two short lengths of pipe. When the gas is lit, cold water enters the bottom pipe of the heater, is heated in a coiled cop-

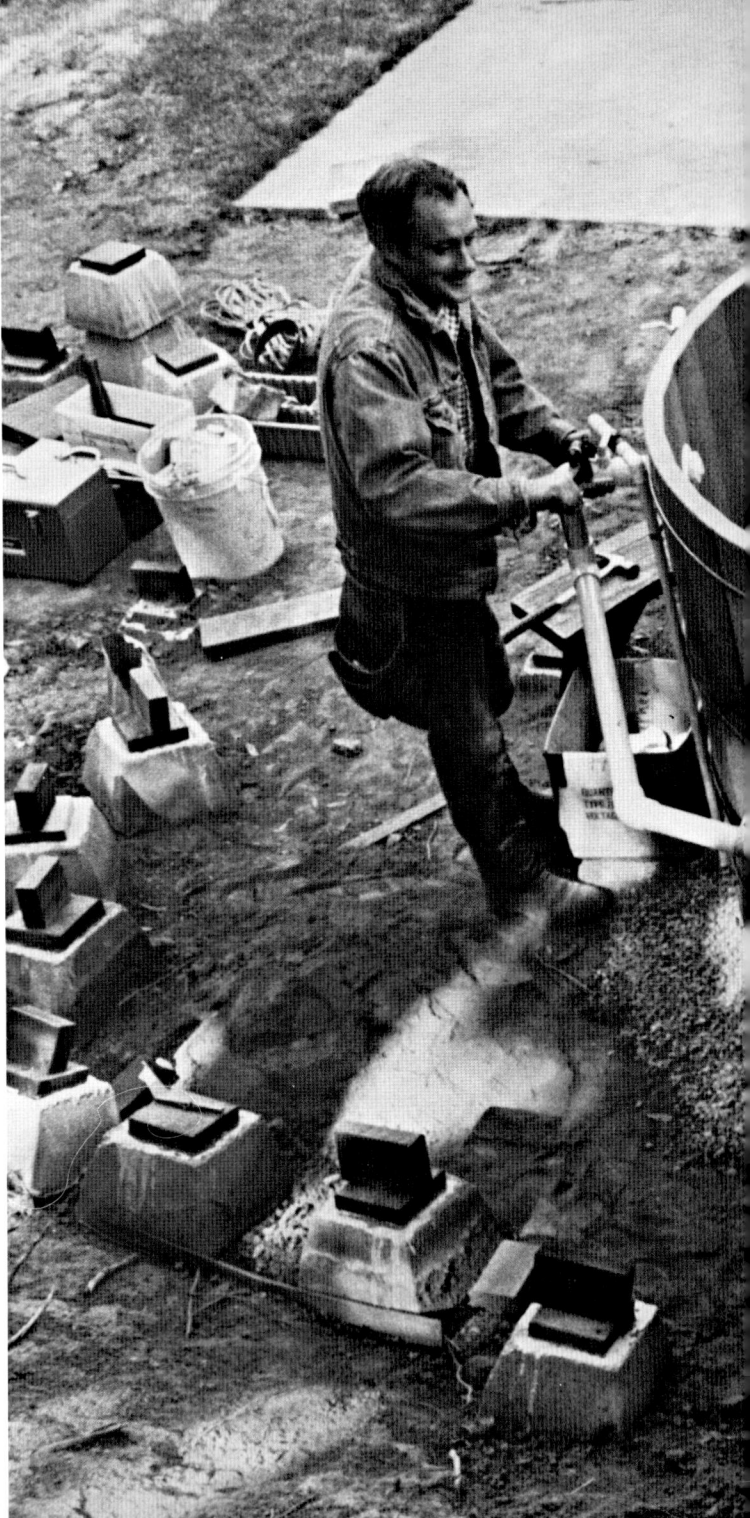

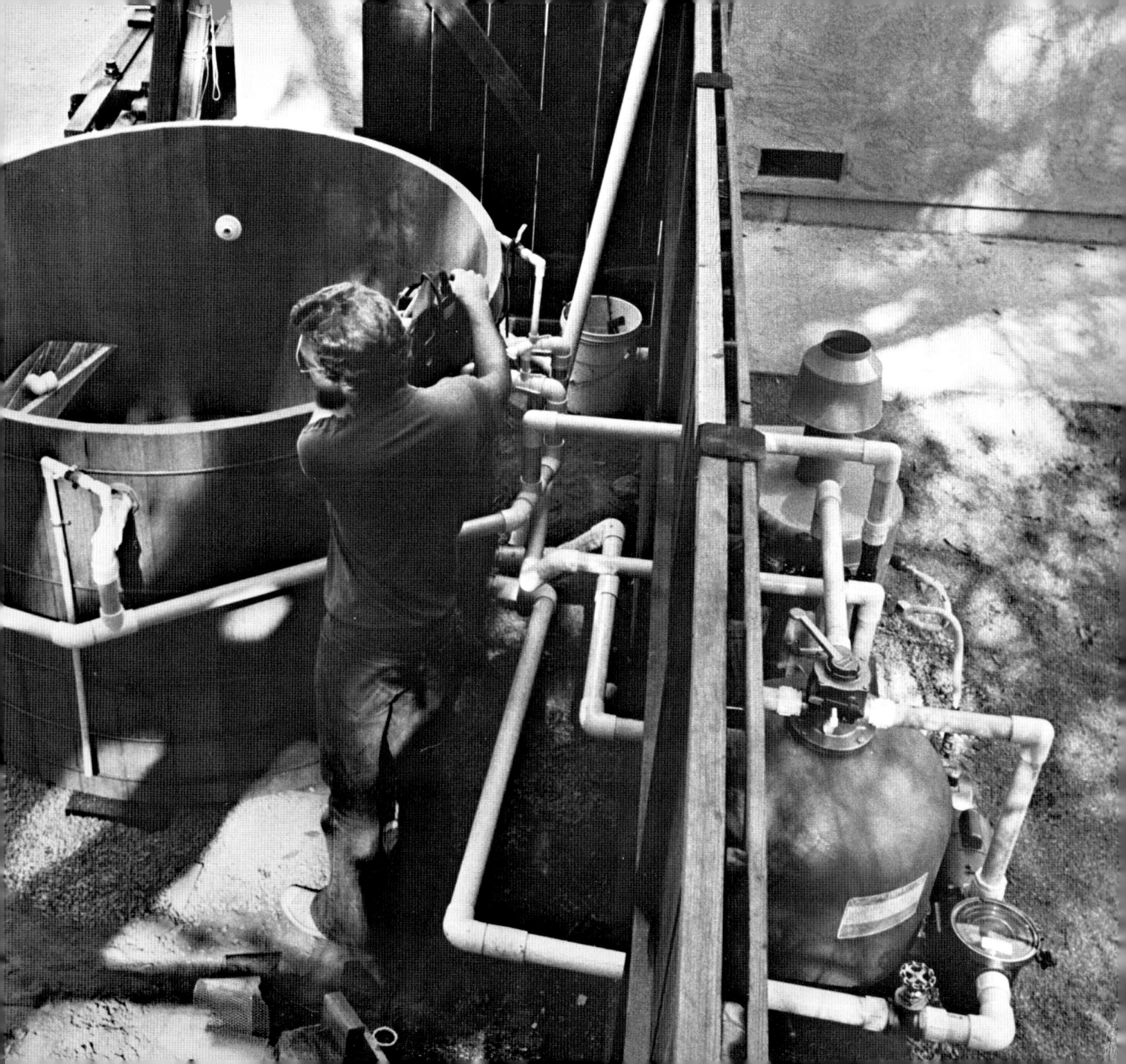

CANNIBAL SOUP

per line over the flame, rises, and enters the tub through the top pipe. This cycle continues until the tub is heated. No pump is required, which makes this heater an energy-saver. A pump is only required for use of the hydromassage system or to circulate the water for filtering purposes. These heaters are equipped with thermostats and deliver around 40,000 BTUs, enough to heat a five-foot tub from tap temperature (5°F.) to 105°F. in four to five hours. Approximately one hour is all that's required to bring the tub to 105° if it was heated the day before.

The filter pictured in this system (previous page) is the permanent-medium type, using sand and gravel. Note the dial valve on the top. Its different positions are explained in the maintenance manual at the end of the book.

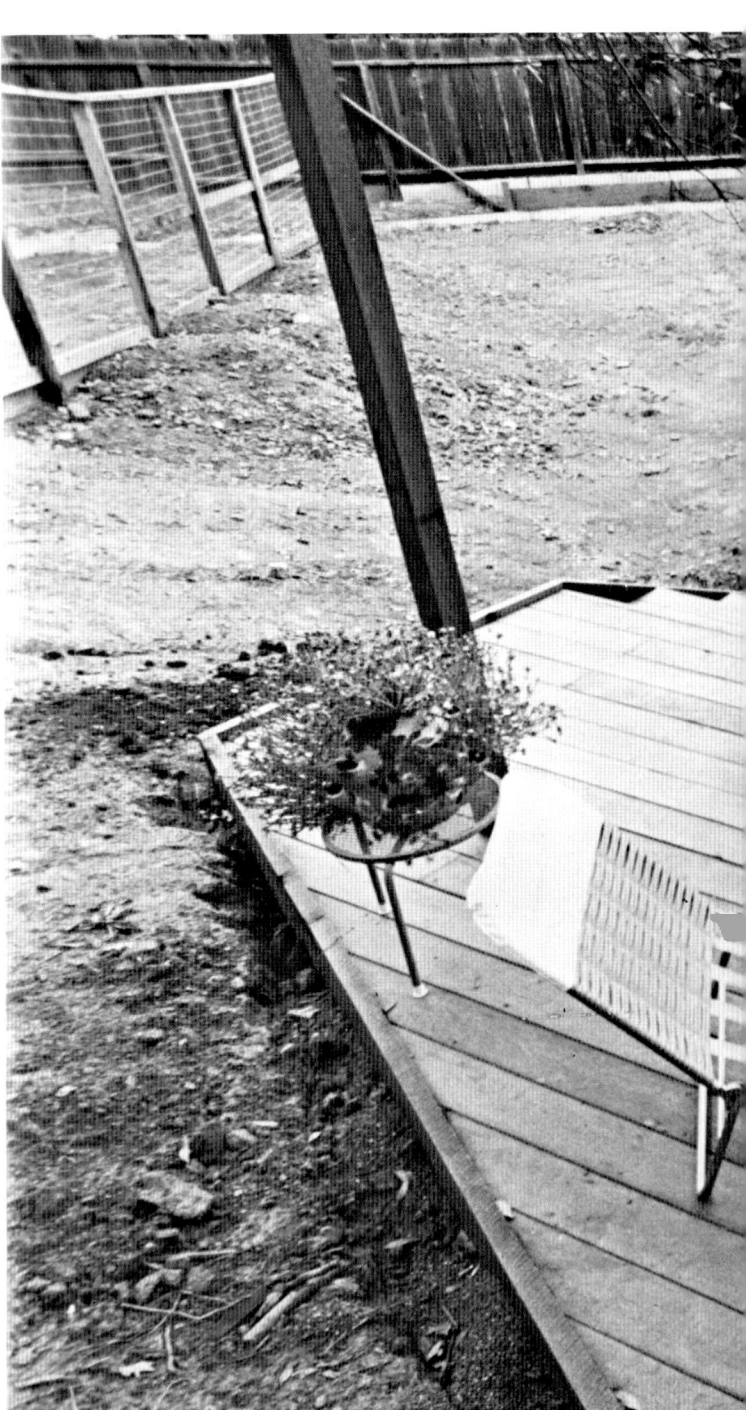

The completed product. This owner chose to have his dealer (Redwood Hot Tubs of Mill Valley, California) install this complicated job. The decking was designed and installed by Warner Yuill-Thorton of Larkspur. The holes in the deck around the perimeter of the tub are for easy access to the hydromassage valves. The redwood cover is halved for ease in handling. Note how well the equipment is hidden behind the fence and shrubbery.

The Parts of Your Tub That Nobody Sees

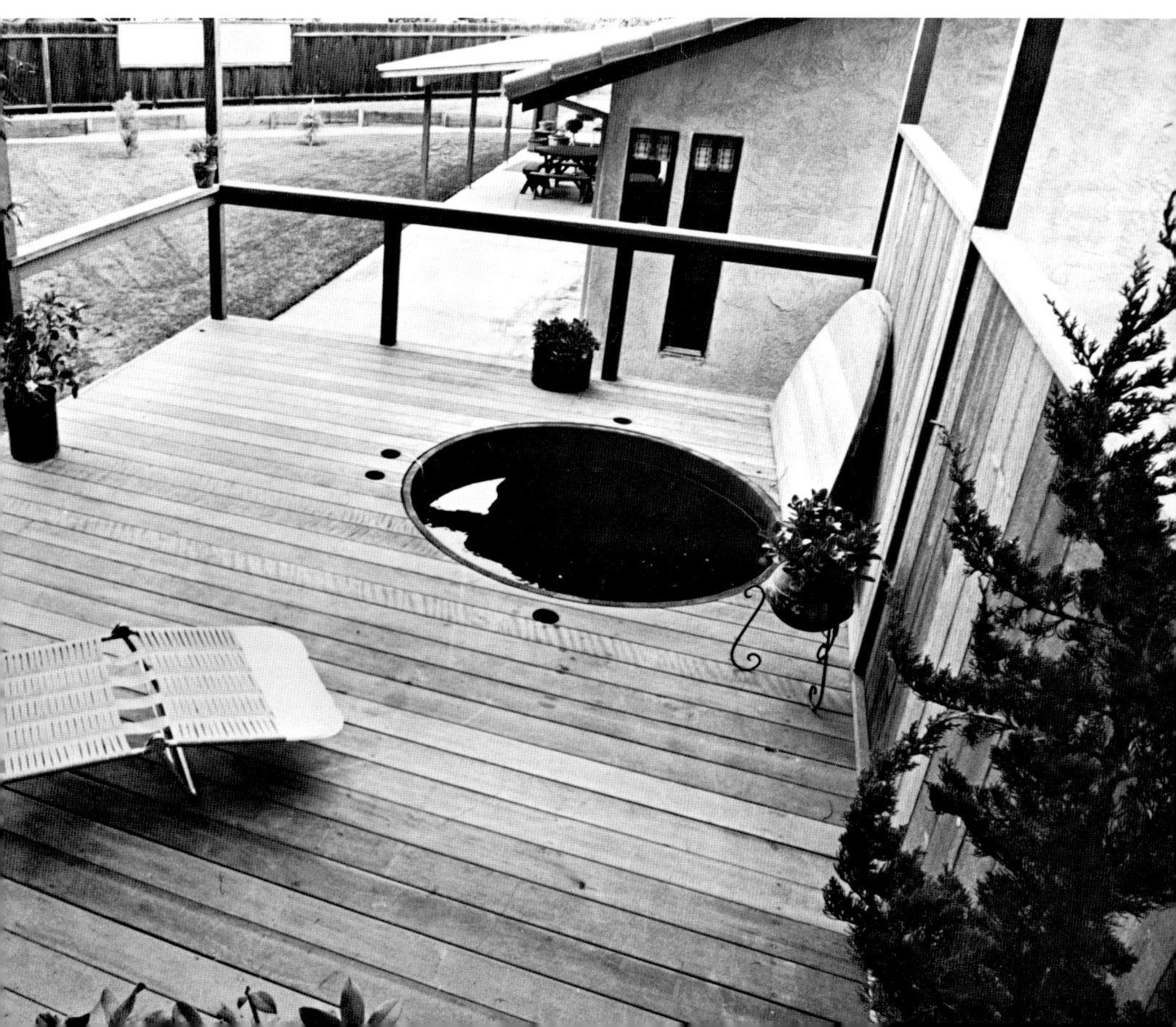

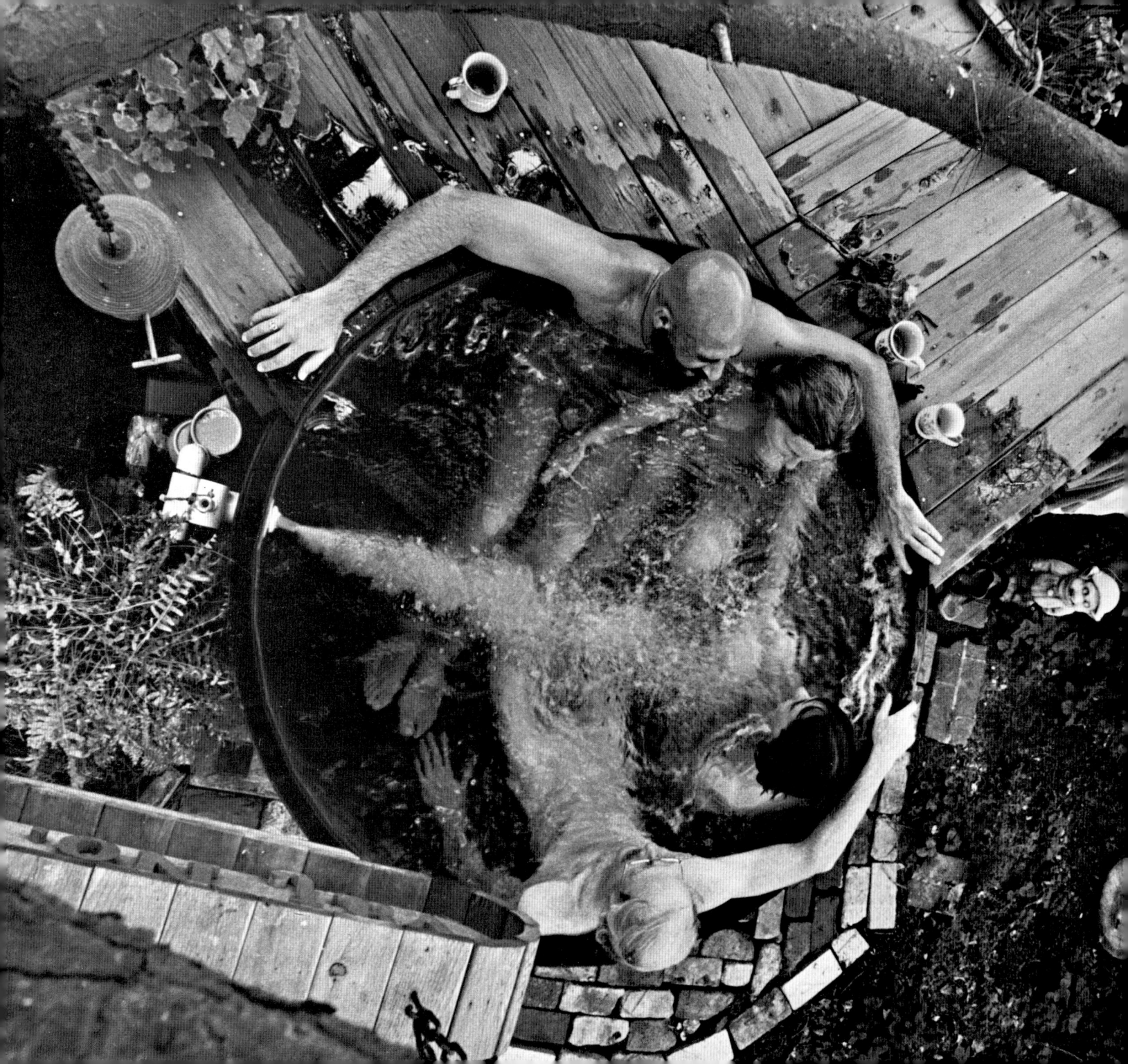

HEATERS AND HYDROMASSAGE UNITS

The heater should be designed specifically for a spa installation to operate at from 100° to 110°F. Flow rate, use time and control sensitivity are important considerations to keep in mind when choosing a heater. You have a choice of two types—electric or gas. Both are similar in operation, but you will find the electric heater takes longer to reach peak heat, which makes it more expensive to operate.

The hydromassage or Jacuzzi jets and plumbing should be matched to the pump's operating capacity. Most dealers use P.V.C. pipe for hooking up the water lines, and most of the equipment is located within ten feet of the tub. The pump, filter and heater are weatherproof, but most tubbers prefer to put a fence around the units or enclose them in a small building. Some hide them under the decking system. Whatever method you choose, be sure to allow adequate ventilation for the heater.

As you can see, there isn't a whole lot to the life support system of your hot tub. If you make sure to buy good equipment, very little maintenance will be required over the years other than standard cleaning and backflushing. So once your equipment is installed and camouflaged to your satisfaction, all that is left to do is climb in and enjoy it.

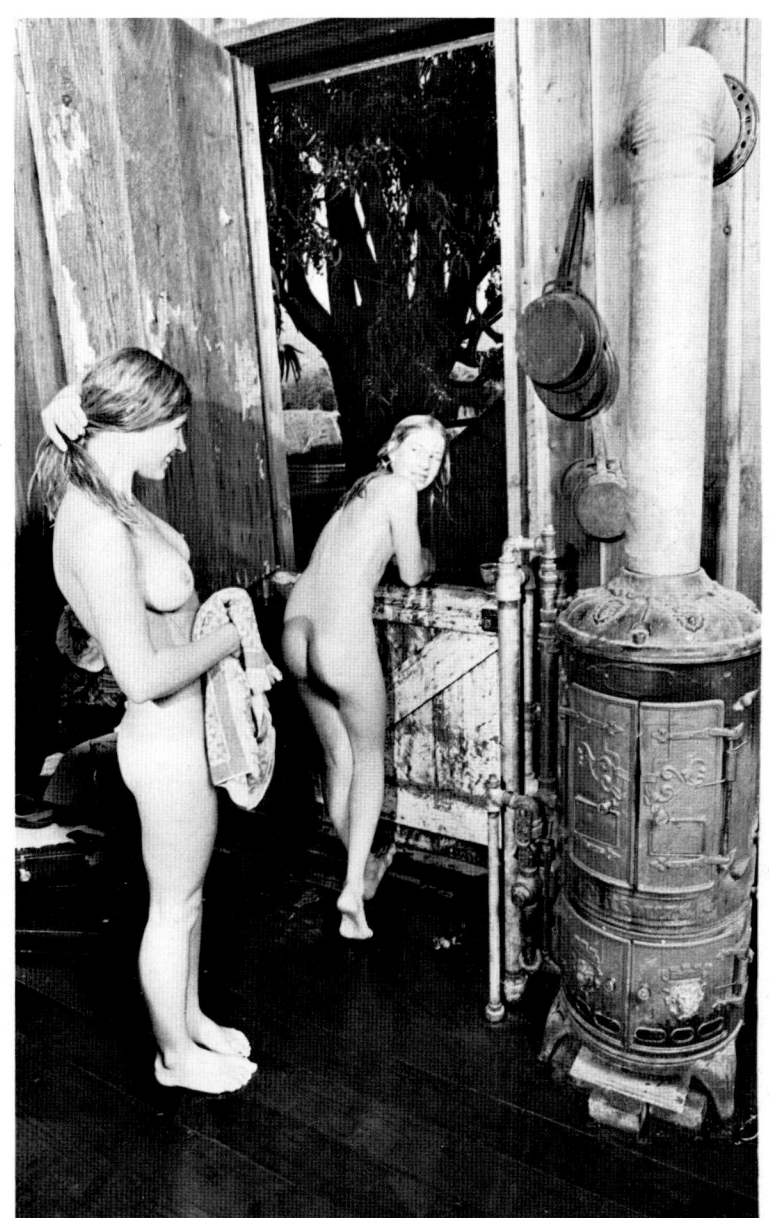

Once used to heat water in a European hotel room, this gas heater makes an attractive hot tub heater. Although good salvaged equipment is hard to come by, if you have it, by all means use it.

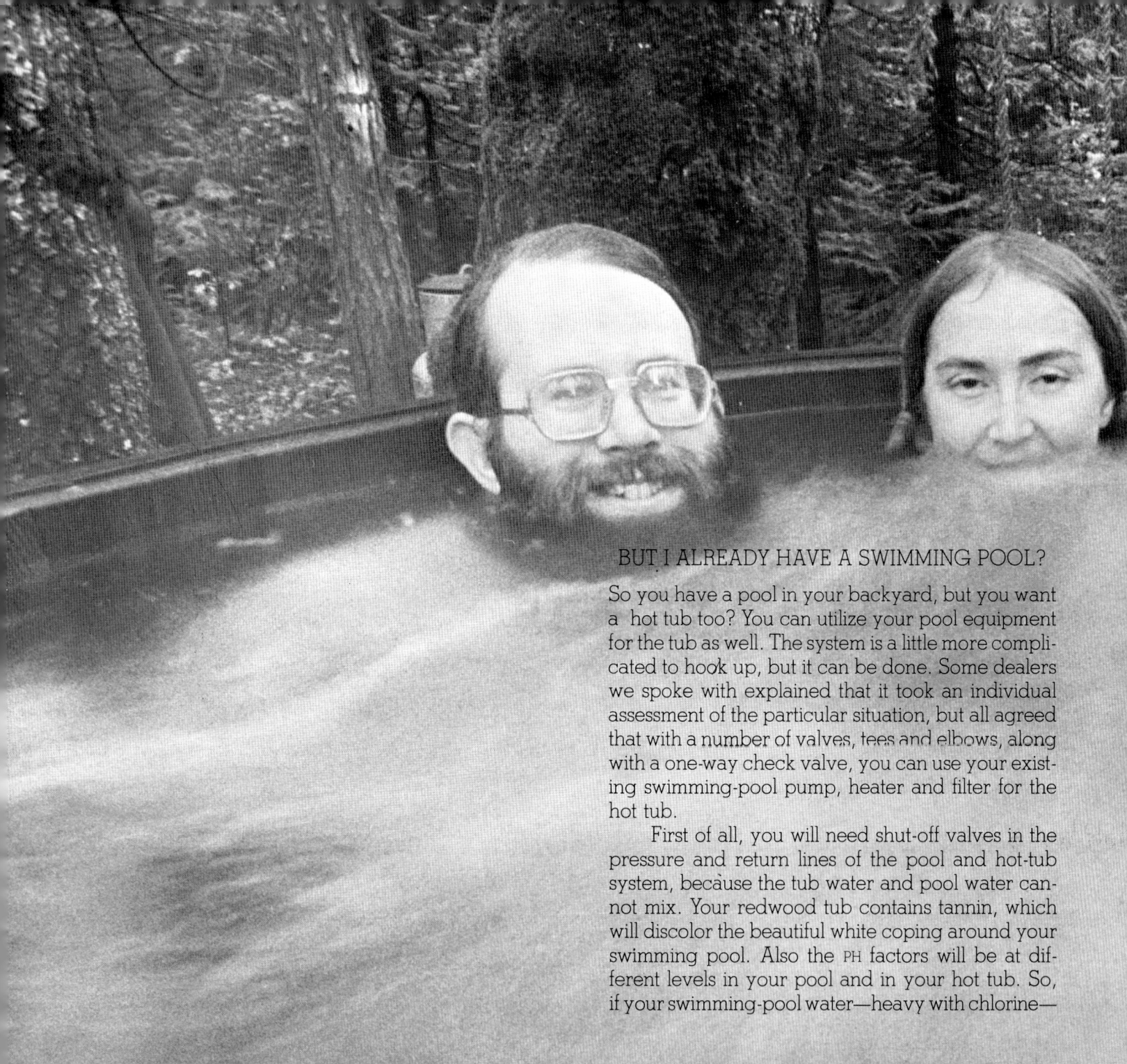

BUT I ALREADY HAVE A SWIMMING POOL?

So you have a pool in your backyard, but you want a hot tub too? You can utilize your pool equipment for the tub as well. The system is a little more complicated to hook up, but it can be done. Some dealers we spoke with explained that it took an individual assessment of the particular situation, but all agreed that with a number of valves, tees and elbows, along with a one-way check valve, you can use your existing swimming-pool pump, heater and filter for the hot tub.

    First of all, you will need shut-off valves in the pressure and return lines of the pool and hot-tub system, because the tub water and pool water cannot mix. Your redwood tub contains tannin, which will discolor the beautiful white coping around your swimming pool. Also the PH factors will be at different levels in your pool and in your hot tub. So, if your swimming-pool water—heavy with chlorine—

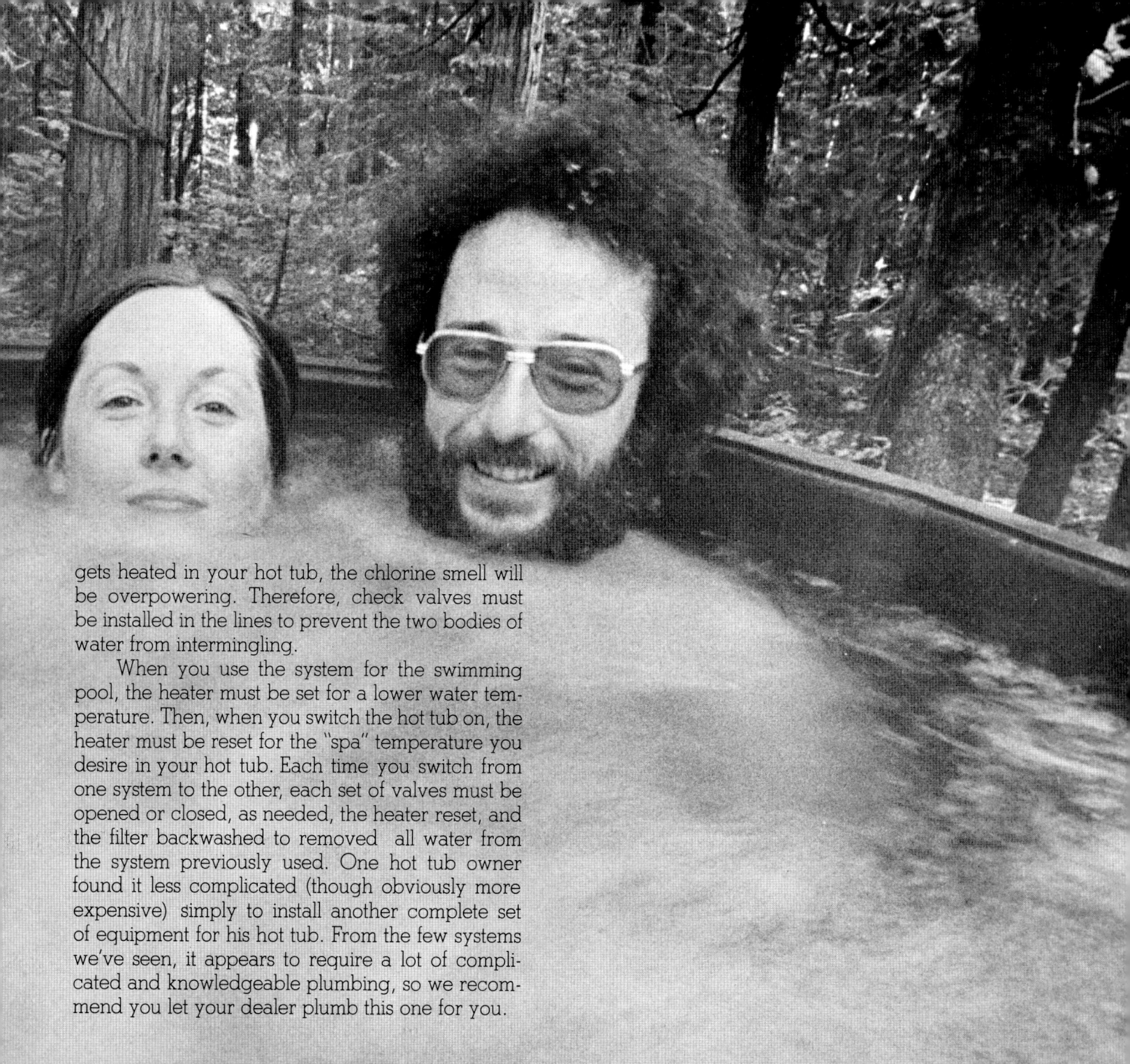

gets heated in your hot tub, the chlorine smell will be overpowering. Therefore, check valves must be installed in the lines to prevent the two bodies of water from intermingling.

When you use the system for the swimming pool, the heater must be set for a lower water temperature. Then, when you switch the hot tub on, the heater must be reset for the "spa" temperature you desire in your hot tub. Each time you switch from one system to the other, each set of valves must be opened or closed, as needed, the heater reset, and the filter backwashed to removed all water from the system previously used. One hot tub owner found it less complicated (though obviously more expensive) simply to install another complete set of equipment for his hot tub. From the few systems we've seen, it appears to require a lot of complicated and knowledgeable plumbing, so we recommend you let your dealer plumb this one for you.

SOLAR HEATING FOR YOUR HOT TUB?

Want to conserve energy? Plug your hot tub into the sun! A five-hundred-gallon tub can be heated to 110°F. with two or three three-by-six foot panels. The solar-heated tub systems we observed were working on a practically maintenance-free basis, and in many cases solar energy was the primary source of heat for the tub.

Your absorbers, or panels, should be located in an area facing south, and preferably slightly higher than the tub itself. The roof of your house or garage might be ideal. To get the maximum direct sun, the panels should be tilted to your exact degree of latitude, plus ten; if your latitude is 35° then tilt the panels 45° and face them south for maximum sun power. (In the southern hemisphere, of course, you would face them north.)

A one-third to one-half horsepower pump is used to keep the water circulating throughout the system, along with a series of relief valves to control thermal expansion. Shut-off valves should be incorporated between each panel for isolation in the event of a leak. Most of the systems we observed were originally installed using P.V.C. pipe in the outlet lines. However, during long periods when the system is not in use, the water temperature in the panels can climb to above 300°F. and melt the outlet pipes. Therefore, many solar engineers recommend the use of copper pipe instead of P.V.C.

We won't discuss solar energy components or products, except to mention that solar companies are springing up all over the country and indicate that solar heating *is* the coming thing. Since it is a relatively new technology please take care in choosing an accredited solar energy company who can help you select the best solar system for your hot tub environment.

If solar heating is within your budget, we recommend this method strongly. Even if you use it only as a secondary source of heat for your tub, you will save money in the long run, and will be participating in conserving precious energy. And in case of brown, grey or black-outs, you'll be able to enjoy your hot tub naturally, with energy from the sun, while millions live by the whims of PG&E or Con-Ed.

In order to receive maximum exposure to the sun, these panels were placed on a nearby hillside. PVC pipe measuring 1½ inches carries the hot water down the hill to the tub where it is picked up by the pump, circulated through the tub and returned to the panels. Since no secondary heating system is used, maximum water temperature on sunny days is 104° F. Try to locate panels as close to the tub as is feasible (on the roof of the house for instance). The greater the distance of the panels from the tub, the greater the heat loss. Note the shut-off valve on the right side of the panel and the check valve on the left.

The Parts of Your Tub That Nobody Sees

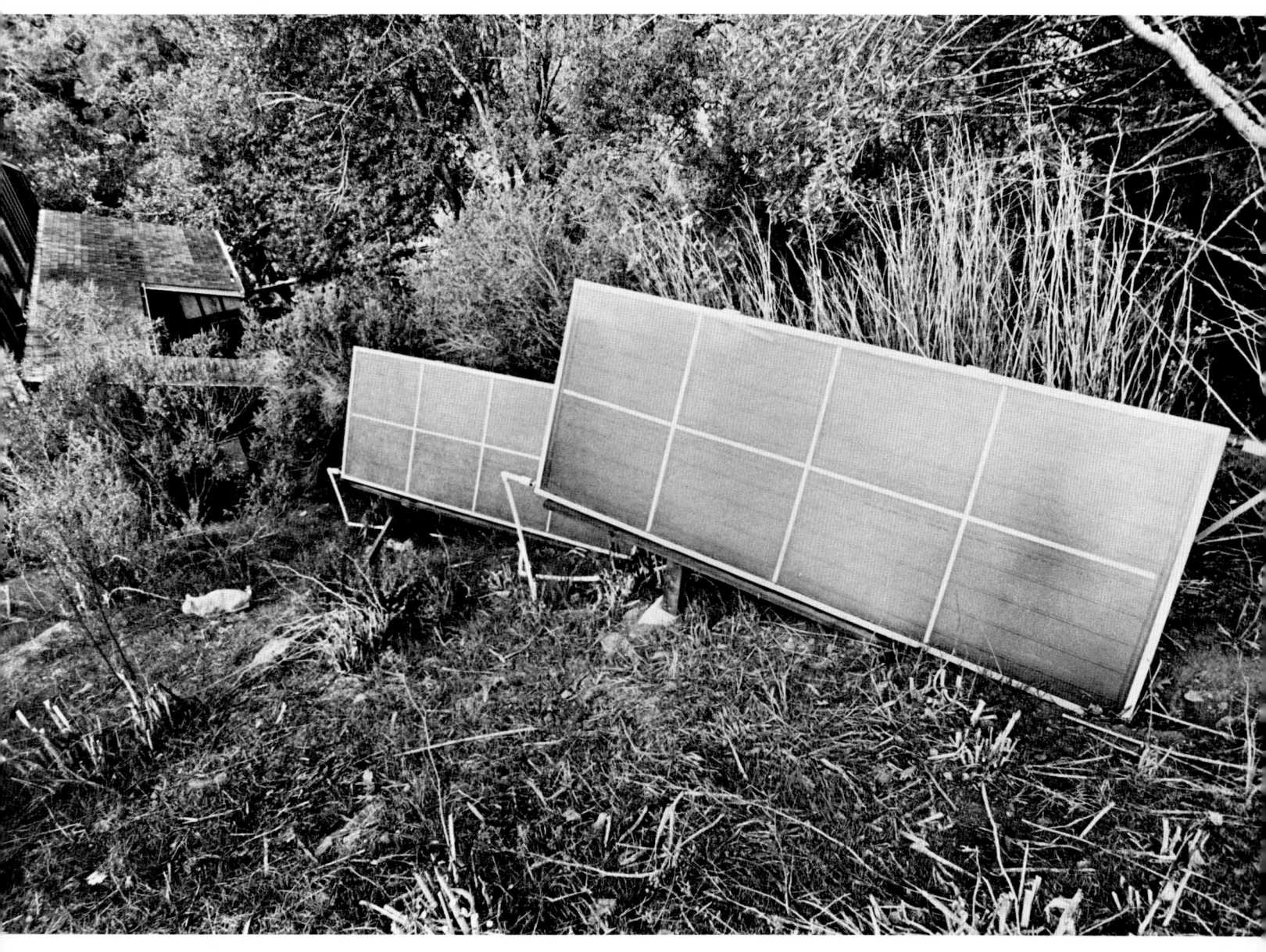

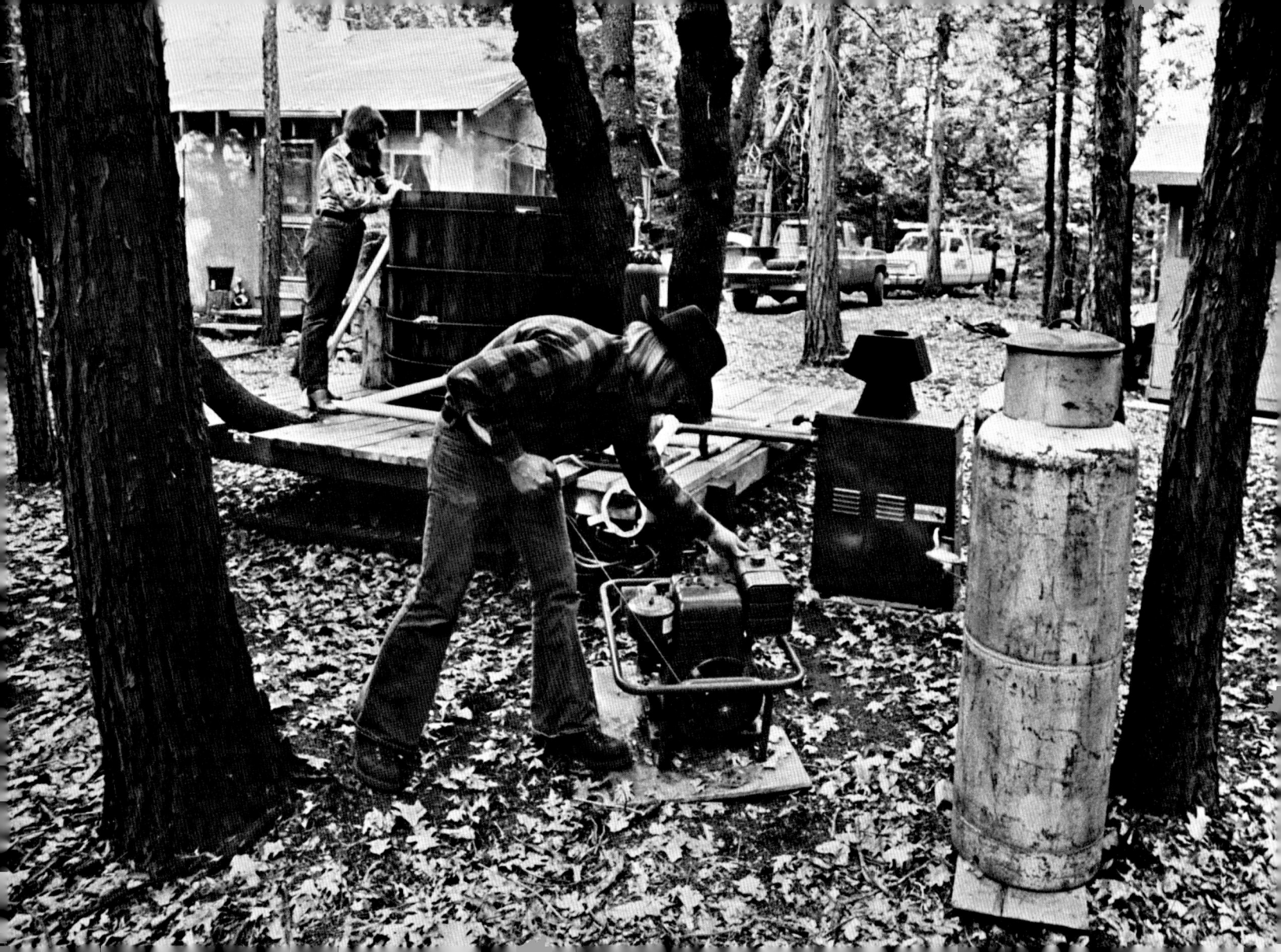

THE THOMPSONS' HOT TUB MAINTENANCE MANUAL

101

Even in remote areas, without the convenience of public utilities, tubbing is possible. The completely self-contained tub shown on the opposite page uses a 4000 KW alternator to run the electric pump, while the heater is fired by a 25-gallon propane bottle.

THE THOMPSONS' HOT TUB MAINTENANCE MANUAL

Your hot tub and its components will require a certain amount of owner maintenance in order to enjoy peak efficiency of your system, but by no means do you need to run out and buy a complete mechanic's toolbox or enroll in a school of engineering. In fact, tools and great mechanical know-how are not really required at all. What is required is a little effort by someone in the family to insure that the chemical balance of the water is maintained, that the filter is clean and operating properly, and that the tub itself is preserved and kept clean. Ninety-nine percent of your time will be spent enjoying the hot tub—one will be devoted to maintenance. Now, those aren't bad odds, are they?

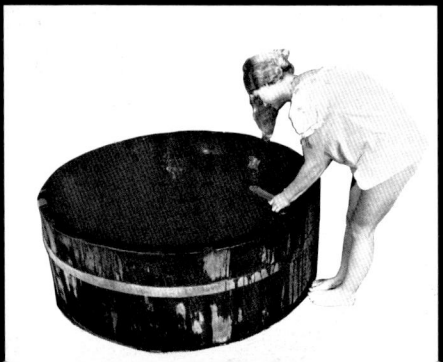

YOUR HOT TUB'S FIRST DAY HOME

When your tub is installed, it must be treated with preservatives or linseed oil. In any case, however, some of the tannin from the redwood will seep into the water. It is perfectly harmless, although it makes the water look rusty. After we changed the water in our tub three times, the water remained clear. Some tub companies now offer a bleaching option before your tub is installed, which eliminates the tannin bleeding completely.

If your tub develops a leak or two, don't worry. The natural swelling of the redwood will usually take care of it. But if the leak persists, dump a one-pound-can full of fine sawdust into the tub. The sawdust will filter into the cracks and swell, sealing the leak. The rest of the sawdust will be removed by your filter.

Coat the outside of your hot tub with linseed oil about once a year. This not only helps preserve the wood, but keeps the steel bands rust-free as well.

In the summer, a styrofoam floating cover is all you need to keep the water warm. In winter use a wood cover for extra insulation. Place the wooden cover flat-side down for better heat control, and flat-side up to provide a vented cover for prolonged periods of non-use. A half-lid, flat-side up, makes a good tabletop for beverages. Both types of covers should be secured when you're away from home so that temptation isn't offered to neighborhood children.

CHEMICALS

The proper use of chemicals is necessary to provide clean, sanitary water; to prevent the spread of bacteria; and to control the growth of algae. Chlorine is the most commonly used chemical to combat these problems. Either dry or liquid form should be added as needed. How much and often it is added depends upon the size of your tub; on how often you use it; and on the temperature level you maintain. The hotter the water, the more often you need to add chlorine.

For example, we have a five-by-four foot tub that we keep at 106°F. and run approximately one or two hours a day. We use four shot glasses of chlorine a week. You need to have a chlorination/alkalinity kit which your dealer may provide, or you can buy one in any pool supply store for around four dollars. Test your water at least every other day.

It is important that the correct level of acidity or alkalinity of the water be maintained. This is what is known as the PH of the water. On your test kit you will find a PH of 7.0 is neutral. Readings above 7.0 are alkaline and readings below are acidic. A desirable range is 7.2 to 7.4. As chlorine is added, it tends to turn the water alkaline, so muriatic acid must be added to maintain proper PH factor. In this range of 7.2 to 7.4 the chlorine is more effective and the cost of the muriatic acid is more than offset by the savings in chlorine.

In our tub, we add a shot glass of muriatic acid once a month. (*Caution: muriatic acid is highly toxic and will burn the skin and eyes severely.*) We mention using a shot glass as a measuring tool. There are no set standards—some use a measuring cup, some a beer bottle, and one owner simply measures by "glugs." Three glugs of chlorine a week and one glug of acid a month.

Whatever works best, but you will find if you maintain the proper PH in your tub and replace what little water you lose from back-washing and evaporation, you will only have to change the water once or twice a year.

Manufacturers of swimming pool products are beginning to develop spa and hot-tub products. One new product we especially like is Clear Spa, a non-toxic, organic, biodegradable spa-water polisher. When Clear Spa is added to your tub, it gathers the small particles of dust or debris together, making them heavy enough to drop to the bottom of your tub and be removed by the filter. Your hot tub will be all the more inviting with sparkling clear water.

GENERAL OPERATING INSTRUCTIONS

When you switch on the pump, all systems will operate automatically. The heater will maintain the temperature at a pre-set level, according to the spa control knob on the side of the unit. (This feature is not available on small, semiautomatic models.) The "recirculate" position the dial valve allows stronger hydrotherapy action. *Always remember to turn off the power switch before operating the dial valve!*

TO CLEAN THE STRAINER BASKET

Your strainer basket catches hair, leaves and lint, and needs to be cleaned about once a week to insure clear water. It's as easy as one to seven. Here's how:

1. Turn off the power switch.
2. Close the gate valve (if such a valve is installed).
3. Move dial valve to "drain."
4. Open the strainer basket lid and clean the strainer.
5. Be sure the basket container is full of water when the gate valve is opened again.
6. Close the strainer, open the gate valve, move the dial valve to "filter."
7. Turn on the power switch and hop in!

To supplement your strainer basket when large leaves or debris fall into your tub, simply use a colander or a strainer with a handle on it. One tub-

THE THOMPSONS' HOT TUB MAINTENANCE MANUAL

ber we know uses a fishnet to scoop the debris.

TO CLEAN THE FILTER

As a general rule of thumb, a permanent medium filter should be backwashed or cleaned once a month. You can determine if your filter needs cleaning by viewing the clear plastic indicator on the side of the dial valve. When the small black float appears in the indicator, it means you *must* clean the filter immediately, because it's becoming clogged. So:

1. Turn off the power switch.
2. Move dial to "backwash" position and attach a garden hose to drain fitting. (Use this water to soak your shrubs.)
3. Turn on the power switch and operate for two-to-five minutes, or until the flow indicator becomes clear.
4. Turn off the power switch, move dial valve back to "filter."
5. Turn on power switch and check the backwash indicator to see that it is now clear.

The cartridge and diatomaceous earth filters are cleaned by removing them and rinsing them with water. Be sure to replace the filters properly in order not to restrict the flow.

TO DRAIN THE TUB

To drain your tub (because of the rusty tannin water or for the semi-annual cleaning) all you do is:

1. Turn the hot tub power switch off.
2. Move the dial valve on top of the filter to "drain."
3. Attach your gardenhose to the drain fitting.
4. Turn the power switch on and drain the tub.
5. Water your yard. The little bit of chlorine left in the water doesn't seem to hurt the plants. After the tub is pumped dry, rinse it with a little fresh water, then allow it to sit empty in the sunshine a few hours before refilling. There is no better disinfectant than the sun.

Then fill the tub with water and add the chlorine. The faint chlorine smell is annoying, but it can be disguised by adding the essence of pine, wintergreen, lemon, herbs, or some of those mineral salts on the market. These additives will have to be repeated every few days, as the filter system removes them.

TO RESTART THE TUB

After cleaning your tub and refilling it with cold water:

1. Turn the dial valve to "recirculate."
2. Turn the power switch on for one minute; then turn the switch off.
3. While pump is on "recirculate," check to make sure *water* is flowing from the air jets—not just air.
4. With switch off, move dial valve to "filter" and leave on until water is heated.
5. Add some chlorine, pine salts and climb in—you've earned it!

HOW YOUR HOT TUB SAVES WATER

At a time when water is scarce in some parts of the country (especially ours) we'd like to point out that a hot tub is not an extravagant water-user. Our five-by-four tub holds five-hundred gallons. That figure may seem excessive at first, but hold on a minute. We found that a hot tub is actually a *water miser*. According to the Marin Municipal Water District in California, each shower you take uses approximately six gallons a minute. The average shower takes approximately seven minutes, and uses forty-two gallons of water. Thus, an average family of four uses up to 168 gallons of water *per day* for showers. Just three days of showering would fill your hot tub at this rate. Or, to put it another way, the amount of water used to fill your tub is equal to fifty minutes of outdoor watering, or ten loads in your washing machine. And, remember, those gallons which fill your tub are not gallons of water that rush down the drain wasted. You only replace that water *once or twice a year!*

For the shower-a-day addict, an invigorating soak in your hot tub instead of a long shower can save you as much as forty-two gallons a day; and for the bathtub user thirty-six gallons. If your mate or family joins you—168 gallons will be saved. We're not saying the hot tub should be used as total substitute for the bathtub, but it does provide an enjoyable water-saving alternative.

Our method: just rinse off with a little water from a hand-held shower attachment, clean with a *loofa* sponge, and then soak in the hot tub, while recirculating the water. (Remember— *never* use soap in your tub.) A *loofa* is such an excellent way to clean yourself in the hot tub that you don't need soap. These natural sponges clean and stimulate circulation at the same time. You can buy a *loofa* in any health food store or bath shop. This way you can relax in your hot tub, massage all over and get completely clean, without turning your shower on. You can also enjoy water-savings of a whopping 4,800 gallons a month! One friend, who has been utilizing the hot-tub bathing method, is contemplating turning his shower stall into an atrium.

The hot tub saves on gas and electricity too! The average single shower uses two thousand BTU to heat the water, thus a family of four uses eight thousand BTU per day for showers. Your hot tub uses only twenty-five hundred BTU per day, so you are therefore not only helping to conserve water by substituting the hot tub for some of your showers, but you are saving gas and money as well!

We hope that this book has been informative and entertaining. We have tried to answer your questions, as well as to pique your curiosity and imagination. Redwood hot tubs are here to stay, as evidenced by the enthusiastic response of tubbers we met while researching and photographing this book. *"We couldn't live without it,"* and *"I never knew anything could feel so great,"* were two heartfelt endorsements we encountered while traveling through Hot Tub Country. The word is out and is spreading fast: Get yourself into hot water.

HAPPY TUBBING, AMERICA!

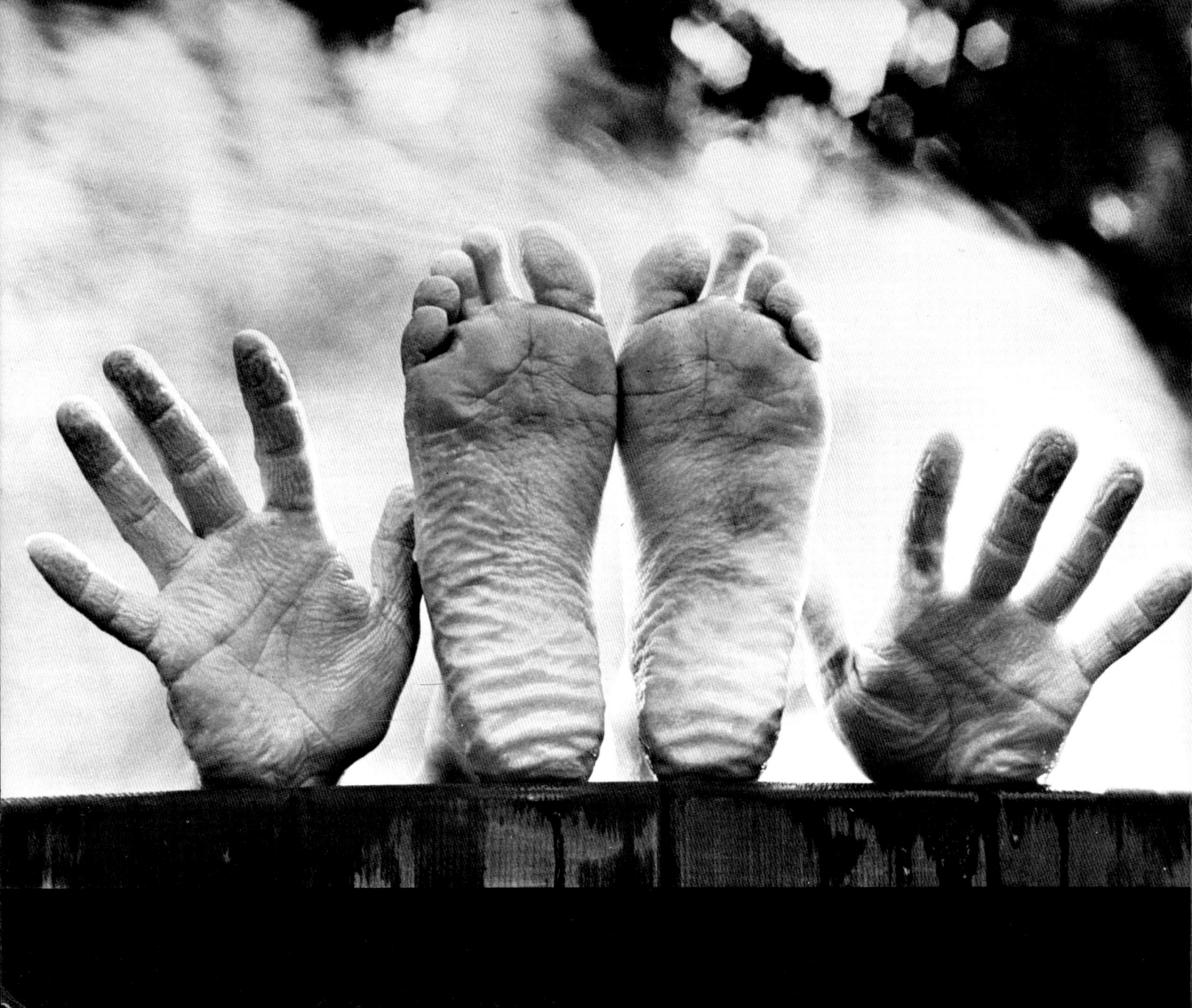

ACKNOWLEDGEMENTS

Tim Wingard
Designer-Contractor
4756 Latigo Canyon
Malibu, California

Leon Elder
Author, *Hot Tubs*
Capra Press
Santa Barbara, California

Allen Lissauer
Redwood Hot Tubs
227 Shoreline Highway
Mill Valley, California

Guy Hadley
International Hot Tubs
5729 Sutter Avenue
Carmichael, California

Allen Krebs
Spring Mountain Hot Tubs
2617 San Pablo Avenue
Berkeley, California

Forrest Allen
Mountain Hot Tubs
P.O. Box 20084
San Jose, California

Gary Gordon & Richard Grant
Gordon & Grant Redwood Tanks
423 Number Quarantina
Santa Barbara, California

Cary Nosler
Health & Nutrition Expert
KCRA Television
Sacramento, California

David Koenigshofer
Koenigshofer Engineers, Energy Consultants
1842 – Eighth Avenue
Sacramento, California

A WORD FROM BEHIND THE SHUTTER

When I started this project I was interested in redwood hot tubs, but I'd never actually been in one. After all these months and these thousands of miles on the road—as people opened their homes and fired up their tubs so we could take the photographs presented here—I've come to two conclusions:

First—either only warm and open people own redwood hot tubs, or hot tubs make very warm and open people.

Second—*I have to have one.* Between photographic assignments, I'm in the process of installing my own redwood hot tub *now*.

I used Nikon 35 mm. equipment throughout the book with Nikkor lenses measuring 18 through 200 mm.

George D. Lepp
Photographer

CANNIBAL SOUP
was printed by the
Mastercraft Press in San Francisco
on Warren's Flokote as four-color
process and monotone. Composition
by San Francisco Design & Type
Studio in Stymie Light.
Book design by Brenton Beck.
Text and picture editing
by Jane Vandenburgh.
Production by R. C. Schuettge
and binding by Cardoza-James
in San Francisco.